The Best Guide
to Allergy

The Best Guide to Allergy

Allan V. Giannini, M.D.

Nathan D. Schultz, M.D.

Terrance T. Chang, M.D.

Diane C. Wong

Illustrated by
Maryanne Regal Hoburg

Appleton-Century-Crofts/New York

NOTICE: The authors and publisher of this book have, as far as it is possible to do so, taken care to make certain that recommendations regarding treatment and use of drugs are correct and compatible with the standards generally accepted at the time of publication. However, knowledge in allergy is constantly changing. As new information becomes available, changes in treatment and in the use of drugs may become necessary. The reader is urged to consult his or her physician for professional advice in dealing with any serious or potentially serious allergic problem.

Copyright © 1981 by APPLETON-CENTURY-CROFTS
A Publishing Division of Prentice-Hall, Inc.

81 82 83 84 85 / 10 9 8 7 6 5 4 3 2 1

Prentice-Hall International, Inc., London
Prentice-Hall of Australia, Pty. Ltd., Sydney
Prentice-Hall of India Private Limited, New Delhi
Prentice-Hall of Japan, Inc., Tokyo
Prentice-Hall of Southeast Asia (Pte.) Ltd., Singapore
Whitehall Books Ltd., Wellington, New Zealand

Library of Congress Cataloging in Publication Data
Main entry under title:

The best guide to allergy.

   (Appleton consumer health guides)
   Bibliography: p.
   Includes index.
   1. Allergy. I. Giannini, Allan V., 1941-
II. Series. [DNLM: 1. Allergy and immunology —
Popular works. WD 300 B561]
RC584.B45   616.97   80-26492
ISBN 0-8385-0645-3
ISBN 0-8385-0644-5 pbk.

Text Design: Judith F. Warm
Cover Design: Lawrence Daniels & Friends, Inc.

PRINTED IN THE UNITED STATES OF AMERICA

*we dedicate this book
to our teachers*

*WILLIAM C. DEAMER, M.D.
OSCAR L. FRICK, M.D.*

Contents

Preface

The Best Guide to Allergy takes you on an updated and authoritative journey over the sometimes mysterious and puzzling backroads of allergy. These backroads must become clearly illuminated highways so that you can make rational and correct decisions regarding your health care. This book, then, is written to provide concise and clear answers to the questions most frequently asked about allergy.

The information contained here reflects the current knowledge of allergy and immunology as studied and taught in the major universities and medical schools of the world. Knowledge has always removed mystery and puzzlement; remember that despots kept entire populations enslaved with ignorance.

Allergy has always had a scrim curtain in front of it, so that only sporadic glimpses of information would light up. This has allowed many healers to carry on with their methods "unhampered by knowledge" to quote the words of the always gentlemanly and learned Professor William C. Deamer, M.D. We have raised the scrim so that every reader will clearly understand the concepts that have been developed and have been proven valid since the first skin test was performed at the end of the nineteenth century. In addition, we have identified the boundaries indicating where information is not yet available and research continues. While our steps have avoided excessively technical language, they are supported on established scientific foundations.

We are indeed four authors. Collaboration of style and content in each chapter step resulted in a unique approach. This has allowed for an open and refreshing presentation of the material.

We hope that this guide will help you and those you care for lead a full and enjoyable life with minimal interference from allergic disease.

Throughout the book, brand name medicines are capitalized (Benadryl), whereas generic names of chemical substances are lower cased (diphenhydramine).

Special thanks go to our publisher — in particular to Mr. Robert McGrath, Mr. Douglas Jones, and Ms. Nancy Shenker for their expert and caring attention to our endeavor.

We would also like to acknowledge the professional assistance of Miss Nancy Thompson who was ready at all times to help with the typewritten preparation of the manuscript.

1

What Is Allergy?

What Is Allergy?

Allergy is an abnormal immune response to substances that do not elicit such adverse reactions in normal individuals.

Allergy or Intolerance?

If you are allergic to a substance, you are likely to experience difficulties or reactions when exposed to small amounts, even traces, of that substance. There are even reports of fatalities from the odor of fish! The allergic person is affected by minute quantities of a substance, whereas even large amounts of that substance cause no adverse reaction in nonallergic people. Penicillin is a good example.

Intolerance is an exaggeration of a, frequently experienced reaction. Most antihistamines can cause some drowsiness. If antihistamines make you excessively sleepy, you are intolerant of them, not allergic to them. To help your physician, keep a careful record of any serious adverse reactions you have. With regard to foods, for example, intolerance (diarrhea or gas) can be very uncomfortable, while allergy (anaphylaxis) can be fatal.

Understanding whether any given reaction is allergy or intolerance will help your physician choose an effective or safe drug in the future.

What Are Allergens?

Allergens are substances (usually proteins) that elicit the allergic response. Among the well-recognized allergens are:

Foods: nuts, fish, eggs, milk, chocolate

Inhalant allergens: house dust, molds, cat and dog dander, pollen from trees, weeds and grasses

Contact allergens: poison oak, poison ivy, and nickel (found in jewelry), that can cause allergic reactions in the skin

Drugs: penicillin, sulfa

Insect venoms: honeybee, wasp, yellow jacket, hornet, fire ant

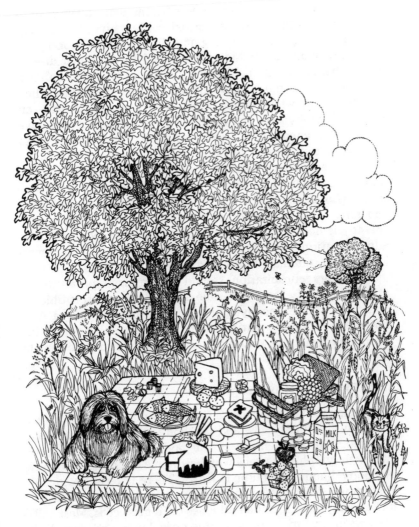

A picnic with allergy.

What Is Anaphylaxis?

Anaphylaxis refers to any type of immediate allergic reaction. The reaction may be limited — a few hives — or it may be generalized, with wheezing and shock (loss of blood pressure). Many agents, including drugs and foods, may cause an acute allergic reaction. Penicillin is the most common drug offender and is much more likely to cause problems when injected than when taken orally. The stings of insects can result in anaphylaxis, and even our most careful patients have unwittingly encountered severe difficulty by eating cookies containing nuts which were not labeled as such.

Many deaths have resulted from untreated, severe anaphylaxis. Mild limited reactions can be treated with antihistamines (for example, Benadryl, Chlor-Trimeton), but severe, generalized reactions require adrenalin by injection. Oxygen therapy is necessary when breathing is obstructed. Cortisone administration prevents recurrence when the offending agent is expected to remain in the body for hours or days.

An allergy consultation should be arranged promptly in order to identify the responsible agent. Persons susceptible to recurrent, severe anaphylactic reactions should carry a life-saving kit containing antihistamines and injectable adrenalin. Your physician can prescribe the kit and instruct you in its use.

What Exactly Is Happening?

The basic mechanism involves four elements: the allergen, the antibody, the mast cells, and the body organs which become affected. The allergen enters the body and comes into contact with lymphocyte cells which produce the primary allergy antibody immunoglobulin E (IgE). There is recent evidence that other classes of antibodies may play minor roles in the allergic response. IgE then attaches onto mast cells. Mast cells are present in various organs — the nose, lungs, and skin. With subsequent exposures to the allergen, the sensitized mast cell becomes excited and releases chemicals, such as histamine and slow-reacting substance of anaphylaxis (SRSA), which are circulated through the body and trigger the allergic symptoms.

SENSITIZATION AND THE ALLERGIC RESPONSE

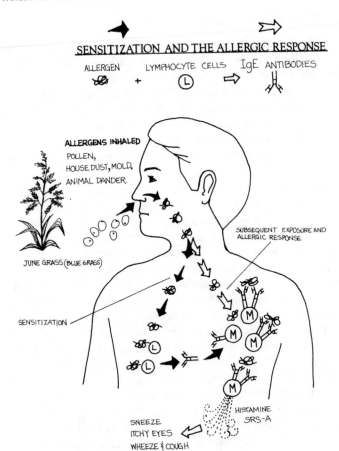

ALLERGEN   LYMPHOCYTE CELLS   IgE ANTIBODIES

ALLERGENS INHALED
POLLEN,
HOUSE DUST, MOLD,
ANIMAL DANDER.

JUNE GRASS (BLUE GRASS)

SENSITIZATION

SUBSEQUENT EXPOSURE AND
ALLERGIC RESPONSE

HISTAMINE
SRS-A

SNEEZE
ITCHY EYES
WHEEZE & COUGH

MAST CELLS RELEASE CHEMICAL MEDIATORS

MAST CELL WITH IgE + ALLERGEN = MEDIATOR RELEASE AND THE ALLERGIC RESPONSE.

        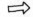

ORGAN RESPONSE
NOSE → ITCH, RUNNY
EYES → RED, WATERY, ITCH
LUNGS → WHEEZE & COUGH

Sensitization and the allergic response.

What Is Clinical Immunology?

The field of clinical immunology is closely allied with the study of allergy as both fields study and treat the immune system. *Immunity* means the ability of the body to protect itself from foreign substances. If we had no immunity, other living cells and viruses would invade our bodies; germs, fungi, and parasites would soon destroy our tissues. An amazing biological phenomenon is the ability of the human body to recognize its own cells while rejecting and killing foreign cells.

Immune protection comes from white blood cells called *lymphocytes.* There are two types, T lymphocytes and B lymphocytes. T cells surround and kill invading bacteria, viruses, and foreign-tissue graft cells by releasing toxic substances. T cells also secrete factors which recruit other types of white blood cells to destroy the foreign substances.

B lymphocytes secrete soluble proteins called *antibodies.* Antibodies have the ability to recognize foreign proteins and other infecting agents. The antibody matches its foe with a submicroscopic mirror image. First, the antibody finds the germs or virus. Once combined with antibody, germs can be more easily ingested by white blood cells or destroyed by the antibody protein called *complement.*

Antibodies are divided into several classes that are all found in serum and are commonly called *gamma globulin.* The most common gamma globulin is immunoglobulin G (IgG), which is responsible for long-lasting protection after vaccinations, such as for tetanus. Immunoglobulin M (IgM) provides rapid but short-lasting protection from infection. Immunoglobulin A (IgA) is present in the blood and is also secreted in nasal and gastric secretions and breast milk. IgA thus provides the first line of antibody defense. Finally, IgE is the primary allergy antibody; most people produce IgE. This antibody provides protection — especially against parasites. An abnormal overproduction of IgE leads to the allergic response.

Clinical immunologists care for people who have deficiencies of the immune system. Immune diseases are often devastating and can be fatal. Patients who do not produce adequate antibodies suffer from recurrent severe infections, and those whose T lymphocytes are deficient are especially susceptible to viral infections and cancer. T lymphocytes can kill tumor cells as well as the cells of transplanted organs; clinical immunologists, therefore, are active in cancer research and work closely with transplant surgeons.

Which Disorders Are Caused by Allergies?

Hayfever, asthma, hives, and eczema are clinical disorders that may be caused by allergies. At times there are also associated complaints which may include stomach aches, headaches, leg pains, excessive fatigue and irritability, pallor, and dark circles under the eyes. Cases of enuresis (bed wetting) have been reported in association with allergy.

How Common Is Allergy?

Latest statistics report that there are 36 million Americans with allergies; this represents 17 percent of our population. Allergy is one of the most common health problems, and everyone knows someone who suffers from allergy. There are 9 million asthmatics in this country. Almost 15 million have hayfever alone, and another 12 million have other allergic diseases. Another way of looking at this is that about one out of every five persons has an allergy.

Other countries report variable differences in the prevalence of allergy, which may reflect racial (genetic) differences.

How Can I Tell If I Have an Allergy?

Classically, allergy is manifested by an immediate, acute reaction to a substance which is inhaled, eaten, touched, or injected. It may also be expressed by more gradually appearing symptoms in the nose, eyes, or chest, such as congestion, itchiness, or wheezing.

A word of caution! These symptoms are not always allergic, and other causes should be considered. Serious infections such as herpes of the eye, parts of toys or food particles lodged in the nose or chest, and infectious bronchitis can all produce symptoms that can masquerade as allergy.

Do Allergic People Catch More Colds?

Yes. Patients with allergy have swelling of their nasal passages and sinus cavities, and manifest infections are easily established when such swellings block the normal drainage of secretions. Serious bacterial infections can develop in paranasal sinus cavities.

Is Allergy Caused By a Virus?

A viral infection can open the door for the development of allergies by acting in several ways. It has been demonstrated in some children that a severe gastrointestinal infection allows food allergens to enter the body more readily through the gut wall and induce the allergic response. A respiratory infection, especially in a child who is genetically predisposed to allergy, may stimulate the development of IgE allergy antibodies.

I've Had My Dogs All My Life.
How Can I Be Allergic to Them?

The ability to have a particular allergy (for example, to dogs) is inherited at birth. You may not manifest this with an allergy symptom such as sneezing or wheezing for many years. Also, you may not have recognized subtle symptoms such as occasional nasal congestion or a slight cough, which are often ignored and taken for granted.

Often, a particular event, such as a viral infection or an excessive exposure to the allergen, will "turn on" your continued allergy response thereafter. Such a triggering event is not always apparent.

Can My Allergies Change over the Years?

Yes, they can. Symptoms may become worse or better; sensitivities to new allergens may develop while previous ones disappear. For example, an infant may have allergic symptoms of eczema and colic from cow's milk and eggs. Within a few years, these food problems can vanish; but they might also be replaced by nasal congestion and sneezing from house dust, molds, or cat dander. Wheezing, along with nasal symptoms, may develop within a short time. If symptoms are worse during the spring, pollen allergy is suspected.

In childhood, spontaneous remission is more common with asthma than with nasal symptoms. Food allergies are usually more of a problem during the early years of life.

Avoidance of your specific allergens over many years may result in the reduction of those sensitivities. Allergy care with skin testing and immunotherapy controls the progression of the allergic state.

How Do Skin Tests Work?

Skin testing is the best practical method of detecting allergens you may be sensitive to. There are two techniques: scratching or pricking the skin and intradermal methods. We initially perform scratch tests; this technique usually reveals the majority of significant allergies. Skin tests by intradermal injection are often necessary when suspected sensitivities are not revealed by the scratch or prick tests.

The purpose is to introduce a small amount of an allergen into the skin. Within a few minutes, the presence or absence of a local reaction of redness or swelling is observed. A significant reaction indicates the presence of the allergy antibody (IgE) to that test allergen.

Which Skin Tests Are the Most Reliable?

Skin tests for specific pollens, animal danders, house dust, and molds are the most reliable and useful. Recently, excellent venom extracts for skin testing for bee sting allergy have become available. Skin tests for foods are sometimes helpful. Finally, testing for an inhalant "chemical allergy" has not been demonstrated to be a valid diagnostic tool.

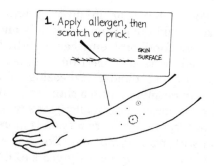

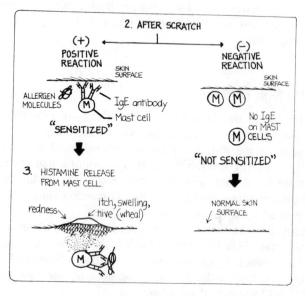

How skin tests work.

Will Skin Tests Tell Me How Severe My Allergies Are?

Only when properly interpreted can allergy skin tests predict the severity of the allergic reaction. Patients who experience more severe symptoms during the ragweed season are likely to have larger reactions. The skin tests are a reflection of the amount of IgE present. Some people with moderate reactions to skin tests and low levels of allergy antibodies may experience severe symptoms because their mucous membranes are unusually sensitive. Occasionally, skin tests are positive when no allergy symptoms are present.

Your allergist must carefully correlate your history and skin test results. Treatment should never be based on skin tests alone.

Can I Have Allergies When All My Tests Are Negative?

Yes. Allergy skin testing is very reliable for animals such as cats; the pollens of grasses, trees, and weeds; house dust; and mold.

The quality of dog extract test material can vary, however. Sometimes the skin test will be negative in a patient who is actually allergic to dogs.

Food skin testing is often misleading. If the food allergy causes an immediate reaction with small amounts, the skin test is usually positive. But if a person is sensitive only to a large amount of the food in question when taken over a prolonged period, the skin test may be negative. Current research points to the digested food products as the actual allergens. We hope that appropriate testing material will be available in the near future.

Antihistamines, especially hydroxysine (Atarax, Marax, Vistaril), may depress the skin test reaction. This could result in a "false negative" test result. All antihistamines should be avoided for 48 hours prior to testing. Steroids (cortisone, prednisone), theophylline preparations (Tedral, aminophylline), and adrenalinlike medicine (Isuprel, Alupent, ephedrine, Brethine) do not affect skin testing and may be used up to the time of this procedure.

Are There Other Tests for Allergy?

Yes, there are. Your allergy specialist can usually tell you about most of your allergy problems without special laboratory tests, but if the problem is complex or puzzling, lab tests may be helpful. Two of these tests are:

1. Microscopic examination for "allergy cells" (*eosinophils*) in the nasal mucus, bronchial secretions, and blood. These cells are commonly elevated in nasal allergies and allergic asthma.

EOSINOPHILS

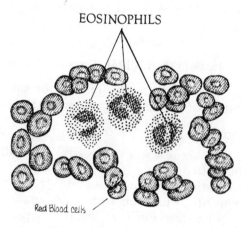

Red Blood cells

"Allergy cells"—eosinophils.

2. RAST (radioallergosorbent test) measures the amount of IgE in the blood. Although this test detects these specific antibodies, it is not as sensitive as skin testing. With RAST testing alone, some allergies may be missed. Moreover, the use of the RAST test has several other limitations, including the number of test allergens available and the high cost. RAST can be helpful with certain food allergies and can clarify the occasional confusing skin test result.

Can Allergy Be Prevented?

The tendency to develop allergies is inherited. Vigorous research in the prevention of allergic disease is being carried out by pediatric allergists in various medical schools. All the answers are not yet in, but several guidelines have become established. Allergic parents-to-be, for example, would be wise to choose breast feeding, which avoids the ingestion of large amounts of allergenic cow's milk protein. Food allergens can even be present in the mother's milk. Nursing mothers of allergic families should avoid eating excessive amounts of such allergenic foods as nuts, chocolate, and eggs (and should perhaps even avoid cow's milk themselves).

The development of specific allergies is related to repeated exposure to the allergens. The presence of animals in the house increases the likelihood of early sensitization. If allergic parents keep a cat or dog in their house, they are asking for trouble.

2
Hayfever

What Is Hayfever?

Hayfever is characterized by an array of symptoms involving the nose, eyes, throat, ears, and skin; these symptoms include nasal congestion, sneezing, and production of clear, watery discharge; conjunctival irritation with watery, itchy eyes; throat soreness and irritation from postnasal drip; ear pains along with the feeling of ear pressure; and generalized fatigue, irritability, and headaches. Hayfever sufferers may have concurrent asthma with wheezing and coughing. The symptoms can occur during a specific season, such as spring, continuously throughout the year, or even sporadically without any pattern.

Hayfever is an old English term originally describing symptoms experienced during hay-pitching time. These symptoms were often so severe that the afflicted person actually felt feverish; hence, the term "hayfever." Now we know that these symptoms are actually induced by grass, which pollinates at hay-pitching time, and not from hay itself. Hayfever is more properly called *allergic rhinoconjunctivitis*.

This condition occurs in individuals who have been previously sensitized by an allergen such as grass pollen. With subsequent exposures, the body's immune system turns on the IgE-producing machinery. The interaction between these antibodies and the allergen(s) leads to allergic hayfever symptoms.

Is Hayfever Seasonal?

Yes, it is. Most persons use the term to refer to clearly defined seasonal difficulties. These usually include nasal congestion, excessive clear nasal secretions, sneezing, itchiness of the nose, watery, itchy eyes, and sometimes itchiness of the ears and throat.

The pollen season varies in different parts of the United States. Ragweed is a severe problem in the East, Midwest and South during the end of the summer. Grass is the strongest allergen in the West, and it pollinates during the months of May and June. Other important allergens which may vary in

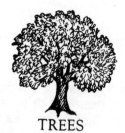

TREES

END OF JANUARY TO END
OF MAY.

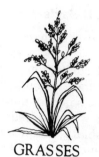

GRASSES

APRIL TO MID OR LATE JUNE.

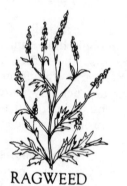

RAGWEED

MID AUGUST TO MID

SEPTEMBER IN THE EAST

AND MIDWEST OF UNITED STATES.

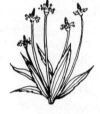

WEEDS

AUGUST TO OCTOBER.

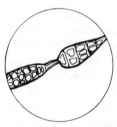 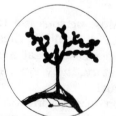

MOLD

SEPTEMBER TO OCTOBER.

The seasons of pollen.

different regions include the pollen of juniper, cedar, and cypress, and the molds *Alternaria* and *Hormodendrum*.

What Is Rose Fever?

"Rose fever" is the folk term for spring hayfever. It originated from the observation that people became congested and sneezed when the roses came into bloom. Actually, the pollen of ornate flowers rarely causes hayfever because it is sticky and does not get into the air. Birds and insects such as bees are attracted to the flowers and carry the sticky pollen away on their bodies to fertilize other flowering plants: thus the meaning of the phrase, "the birds and the bees." If you smell flowers, of course, problems can result. So remember: Hayfever or allergy plants rarely have large, beautiful, or fragrant flowers.

Can I Have Hayfever Symptoms All Year?

Yes. Your symptoms may persist even through the winter months when pollens are no longer present. House dust is the major cause of perennial (year-round) allergic rhinitis. An insect which is best seen with a microscope is the important allergic component of house dust, the house dust mite. The concentration of the house dust mite varies with changes in climate in different cities; nevertheless, the genus is identical throughout the world, *Dermatophagoides* ("skin eater"). It lives on surfaces of mattresses and flooring, but not on people. Of greater interest, however, is the fact that it feeds on the tiny flecks of human skin and animal dander which are constantly shed; thus the biological name.

Animal dander from your cats and dogs is also responsible for your nonseasonal allergies. This is usually the most important cause of allergy in homes with pets.

Finally, mold allergy must be kept in mind, especially in older homes with damp rooms. Other sources are showers, decks, porches, and house plants. Recent studies also point to straw carpets and woven baskets as important sources of mold spores.

Why Can't I Smell?

You are unable to smell when allergies cause severe swelling of the mucosal lining of your nose. The olfactory nerve endings for the sense of smell become blocked by the edema and the excessive secretions so that the tiny molecular particles of food and so on that transmit odor do not make the necessary contact.

After receiving appropriate treatment for nasal allergies, patients are often surprised—and delighted—that they can again smell. Bon appétit!

Do I Have a Cold or Allergy in My Nose?

You may indeed have a cold. If your symptoms persist for months, however, and if there are no other household members with similar complaints, then you probably have a nasal allergy that is masquerading as a cold.

The nasal mucosa — the lining of the nose — is characteristically pale or pearly gray with allergy. With a cold it is red and angry! In addition, the characteristic white blood cells, eosinophils, are often present in the clear allergic nasal secretions.

Finally, patients with untreated allergies are more susceptible to colds. Repeated colds are indeed infections, but they tend to recur because of the underlying allergic state. Once the allergy is under control, so is the exaggerated frequency of such infections.

Why Are My Eyes Red?

Nasal allergies commonly involve the outer membrane of the eye, the *conjunctiva*, which, like your nose, contains mast cells. (Remember, the mast cells release histamine when allergies occur.) The released histamine causes the swelling by allowing leakage of watery fluid into the surrounding eye tissues. It also causes blood vessels in your eyes to dilate, causing the reddish appearance. Rubbing your eyes adds to the redness.

Can Hayfever Cause Nosebleeds?

Nosebleeds can occur as a result of trauma from either rubbing the itch or blowing your nose too often or too hard. Also, as nasal secretions dry, they may pull away and tear blood vessels. Beware of the excessive use of nasal sprays, which can also contribute to the problem. Once bleeding begins, it can easily be stopped by tilting your head back at an 45° angle and applying direct pressure to that side. Call your physician if nosebleeds are persistent.

What About Nasal Sprays?

Over-the-counter medications (such as Afrin, Neo-Synephrine and Dristan) are useful for a short time when nasal symptoms become severe. These sprays work by constricting engorged blood vessels and subsequently shrinking the swollen nasal mucosal tissues, thereby allowing greater movement of air through the nasal passages.

Their immediate effectiveness in controlling your hayfever symptoms might tempt you to continue their usage for prolonged periods. If these sprays are used for more than two or three days consecutively, you cannot expect the same nasal relief that you had initially. The nasal tissues become tolerant of the medication and may actually "rebel" by growing more swollen and red, evolving into a serious condition known as *rhinitis medicamentosa*. Thus, nasal sprays should not be continued for more than 2–3 days at a time unless recommended by your physician.

What Is the Best Medicine for Hayfever?

The best medicine for hayfever is a balanced combination of an antihistamine with a decongestant. The antihistamine blocks the chemical mediator (histamine) released by mast cells and prevents activation of the allergic response. The decongestant directly constricts blood vessels and helps to reverse the allergic symptoms, reducing the redness and itching of the eyes as well as the swelling that causes congestion. Atropinelike drugs also dry excessive secretions.

ANTIHISTAMINE CLASSES: EXAMPLES OF BRANDS

Class I: Ethanolamine
   Benadryl*
   Rondec*

Class II: Ethylenediamine
   Pyribenzamine (PBZ)*
   Triaminic

Class III: Alkylamine (most over-the-counter preparations)
   Chlor-Trimeton (chlorpheniramine)
   ARM
   Allerest
   Teldrin
   Ornade*
   Actifed*
   Copyronil*
   Triaminic

Class IV: Piperazine
   Tacaryl*

Class V: Phenothiazines
   Phenergan*

*Prescription necessary.

Some effective combinations are available without prescription: Triaminic, ARM, and Allerest. Prescription products such as Ornade, PBZ with Ephedrine, and Rondec, which include different chemical groups, are often necessary.

Some people cannot take an antihistamine because of drowsiness, while others cannot tolerate a decongestant because of irritability or difficulty with high blood pressure. In such cases, each drug can be taken separately. Again, some are available and effective without prescription: among others, the antihistamine Chlor-Trimeton and the decongestant Sudafed. Visine and Murine eye drops provide decongestant for eye symptoms. Your physician may also prescribe cortisone for a short time if your symptoms are severe.

Aspirin containing combinations is not necessary and can, in addition, be harmful for asthmatics.

Can I Take Hayfever Medications for a Long Time?

Yes. The antihistamines and decongestants prescribed for hayfever may be taken for many years. Possible side effects, however, should be monitored; these may occur even when the duration of treatment is only a few days.

Certain antihistamines can cause excessive drowsiness and may cause impotence during the course of treatment. Because decongestants can aggravate high blood pressure, they should be used with caution.

At times, short courses of steroids (cortisone or prednisone) may be necessary to control severe symptoms for one or two weeks of the year. This is safe in most cases, but if high doses are continued, severe side effects may occur.

Are There Any New Medicines Available for Hayfever?

New effective medications are available in other countries. These include nasal sprays — cromolyn sodium, beclomethasone, and flunisolide — and are under evaluation for use in the United States.

New brands of antihistamine-decongestant combinations, however, are usually just different variations of the older drugs.

Can Hayfever Lead to Asthma?

Yes. There is evidence that, when untreated, hayfever is likely — but not certain — to lead to allergic asthma. Very often, the symptoms of hayfever are the first signs of allergy, and wheezing subsequently develops. The wheezing sometimes starts when the nasal and eye symptoms become very severe. At other times, the hayfever stops and the asthma becomes the allergic manifestation.

What About Christmas Trees?

Christmas trees cause allergic symptoms in many people. The most common sources of difficulty are the airborne pollens and molds that are in the trees and that remain there after they have been cut down and stored. A person who is sensitive to these pollens and molds will come into close contact with them when a large, moist tree comes into the home. The heat of the house helps to release these inhalant substances into the closed indoor environment, and thus a family recreates a specific pollen or mold season for a few weeks in December.

Recent studies have indicated that a specific allergenic chemical, *terpene*, is released by the tree itself. This substance directly causes allergy symptoms of nasal congestion and discharge and wheezing in a sensitized individual.

Do I Have "Sinus"?

Because they feel fullness in the nasal area, the term "sinus" is frequently used by patients to describe the nasal stuffiness associated with hayfever. The sinuses are cavities with openings to the nasal passages and are lined with membranes similar to those in the nose.

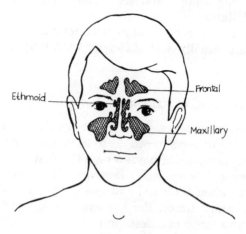

The sinuses.

The medical term *sinusitis* refers to inflammation or infection of the sinuses. When the sinus openings are blocked by the swollen nasal membranes, pressure changes occur and are probably the cause of most recurrent sinus headaches. The often intense pain is relieved by reducing the swelling of the membranes.

Bacterial infections of the sinuses require prompt medical attention. When the sinus openings are blocked and mucus is present, ideal conditions for bacteria are created. Bacterial growth causes the development of pus, which, in turn, pushes against the walls of the closed sinuses, causing pain. This pain is most severe over the sinuses—under the eyes, "behind" the eyes, and in the forehead over the eyes. The pain may also radiate to the back of the head. Yellow or green pus may discharge from the nose or drip into the back of the throat. If the infection goes untreated, the sinus can rupture, pushing bacteria and pus onto the brain, a serious and frequently fatal complication. Proper antibiotics usually resolve the situation promptly. Occasionally, the sinuses must be surgically opened and drained.

What Is Vasomotor Rhinitis?

Rhinitis means inflammation of the nose. Basically, the nasal mucosa can react to the environment in two ways. It can secrete mucus and swell. In some patients, these allergylike symptoms are the results of physical factors, such as temperature change, air pollution, humidity change, or odors; emotions may also play a role. *Vasomotor* refers to the motor control of the blood vessels. This regulates the edema (swelling) and clear secretions of the mucous membranes.

Extreme temperature changes or pollution, such as smoke, can cause almost anyone's nose to become blocked. Vasomotor rhinitis is an exaggerated sensitivity of these factors.

You should suspect vasomotor rhinitis if you develop a stuffy, runny nose, and sneezing when you get out of the shower on a cold morning or when you go outdoors on a smoggy day. Often, vasomotor rhinitis and allergies occur together and an allergy should be investigated. The treatment of vasomotor rhinitis is decongestant medication. These drugs, pseudoephrine or phenylpropanolamine, by any brand names, shrink the membranes and allow you to breathe. They are not curative and only control symptoms. Although they may make high blood pressure worse while you are taking them, decongestants rarely cause drowsiness. Cortisone nasal sprays may be necessary for short exacerbations. Ordinary nasal sprays must be avoided. With time they become habit forming and less effective; this is called *rebound*. The spray medication itself irritates the nose, making the condition worse.

What Is a Deviated Septum?

The bone that devides the nose into the right and left sides — the *septum* — may be closer to one side, narrowing that opening. You may be born with a deviated septum or it may result from injury. When the nasal membranes are swollen from allergy, the obstruction may become more severe, obstructing one side of the nose. Your physician can diagnose a septal deviation by a physical examination of the nose. Surgery can relieve the bothersome obstruction when the deviation is severe.

What Are Nasal Polyps?

Polyps originate in the sinuses. They are formed when a surface of the membrane becomes loaded with fluids and swells. Portions of this membrane bulge out, fill the sinuses, and protrude into the nose, frequently blocking the nasal passages.

Polyps are not tumors or growths, and, moreover, their relation to allergy is disputed. Polyps occasionally disappear, but treatment is usually necessary. Cortisone by nasal spray or intranasal injection may be tried first.

Polyps are a frustration because they frequently recur in spite of all treatment; surgical removal is often required when this is the case. When the lining membranes of the sinuses become continually inflamed, swollen, and infected, the otorhinolaryngologist (ear-nose-and-throat specialist) may need to create new sinus openings and remove some of the diseased membranes.

3
Asthma

Can I Die From Asthma?
When Shall I Call My Physician?
Should I Move?
Can Asthma Be Cured?

What Is Happening in My Chest?

Bronchial asthma is, as the name implies, a disease affecting the bronchial tubes. Air enters the chest through the *trachea*, commonly called the "windpipe." The trachea divides into the right and left mainstem bronchi (bronchial tubes). These tubes themselves divide again and again to form many hundreds of tiny bronchial tubes or *bronchioles*.

In the lining of the bronchial tubes there are mucus-producing cells called *goblet cells*, which are covered with tiny, hairlike fibers called *cilia*. With a beating motion, cilia move mucus from the bronchial tubes through the trachea. In this way the bronchial tubes clean themselves. Strands of muscles encircle the bronchi.

During an attack of asthma, these muscles involuntarily contract, constricting the bronchial tubes. At the same time, the goblet cells produce large amounts of sticky mucus (phlegm). As the chest expands during inhalation, air enters the bronchial tubes on its way to the tiny breathing sacs (*alveoli*) at the ends of the tubes. When the asthmatic tries to exhale, these bronchial tubes become even smaller and air is trapped in the lungs. Air going through the narrowed tubes creates the sound and sensation of wheezing. The mucus forms plugs which narrow some air passages, and close others completely. When air cannot move in and out a person feels short of breath or *dyspneic*. The blood flows through the walls of the alveoli without picking up needed oxygen or giving off carbon dioxide.

Is Asthma Always Allergic?

No. Asthma is *frequently* a result of allergies to animals, dust, pollens, molds, and foods. Sometimes, however, asthma has

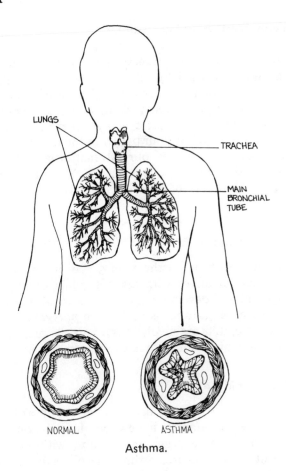

LUNGS

TRACHEA

MAIN
BRONCHIAL
TUBE

NORMAL   ASTHMA

Asthma.

no allergic cause and is only a hypersensitive and highly irritable condition of the bronchial tubes.

How Can I Find Out if My Asthma Is Caused by Allergies?

You should be evaluated by an allergy specialist. This may include skin testing, possible trial elimination diets, and laboratory studies.

Will Allergy Shots Help My Asthma?

Yes. Allergy shots (immunotherapy) can help certain patients whose asthma is caused by allergy to pollens, molds, dust, and even animal danders. Research studies have confirmed that immunotherapy prevents asthma that is secondary to pollens and cats. (Of course, the best treatment for animal allergies is the removal of your pet from the house.)

Allergy shots have helped our asthmatic patients tolerate the spring and summer pollen seasons. They are now also able to visit the homes of friends and relatives who have cats and dogs.

Is Asthma Hereditary?

The tendency toward asthma may be inherited. Many asthmatics have relatives with asthma, while others do not. Environmental and developmental factors are also important. The inheritance of asthma is said to be *polygenic*, meaning that many gene units are involved and must be present in just the right combination for asthma to develop.

Why Asthma at My Age?

Asthma may strike at *any* age: the onset of asthma frequently occurs in infancy; a new pet in the house might trigger asthma in a teenager; commonly, without warning and without allergic cause, asthma develops in the menopausal years. Asthma that develops in childhood may subside only to reappear in later life. Additionally, asthma may occur in an individual who previously had eczema or hayfever.

Does Coughing Trigger Asthma?

Many asthmatics say, "If I could only stop coughing I wouldn't wheeze." They are sometimes correct: postnasal drip and excess mucus irritate the throat or trachea, and the coughing can trigger the spasms of asthma. Conversely, a cough is frequently the first sign of asthma itself. This is true in both children and adults. In such cases, patients cough *because* they are wheezing: they are, in fact, having *bronchospasm*. When the asthma or wheezing is relieved, the cough will subside.

Is Asthma Like Emphysema?

Emphysema and asthma are quite dissimilar. Asthma is, by definition, a reversible or controllable disease; that is, with proper treatment, normal breathing can be restored, at least temporarily. In emphysema, the alveoli are actually destroyed. When the small airways are irreversibly destroyed (often by smoking) the diagnosis of chronic obstructive pulmonary disease (COPD) is made.

There is *no* evidence that asthma leads to COPD or emphysema.

What About Infections and Antibiotics?

Infections can cause asthma. Infections that affect asthma are respiratory infections such as influenza, the common cold, and sinus infections. People with asthma tend to develop respiratory infections more often.

Sinus pains, increased nasal congestion, wheezing, chest tightness, and exacerbation of coughing spells with discolored sputum are symptoms of an infection. These should be recognized together with the familiar general fatigue, headaches, and fever. Always be on the alert for these signs and do everything possible to prevent the buildup of an asthma attack.

When possible, stay away from people with colds and other respiratory illnesses. Keep in mind that being in crowded places during the fall and winter months exposes you to others' infections.

Antibiotics, such as penicillin or tetracycline, may or may not be helpful. Do not be misled by thinking that antibiotics will always cure your infections and asthma. In fact, only infections that are caused by bacteria need to be treated with antibiotics. Colds and influenza are caused by viruses. If you think that an antibiotic is necessary, ask your physician to evaluate the infection and confirm your need for it.

Is Asthma Emotionally Related?

There are undoubtedly some individuals who know that they can make their asthma worse by becoming excited or angry. In these cases, therapy is directed at controlling emotional upsets which can trigger the asthma attacks. Most of the time, however, it is difficult to sort out exactly how important emotions are in causing asthma. As a cause of asthma, emotions have been exaggerated and unnecessarily have become the focus of parental concern. Instead, emotions should be regarded as one of the many possible aggravating factors of asthma which must be equally considered and evaluated by a physician.

Is Biofeedback Helpful?

Stress can trigger wheezing and wheezing creates stress. This cycle must be broken. The various techniques used to break this cycle are collectively called *behavior modification*. Biofeedback and autogenic training are two such techniques under investigation.

If you are able to teach your body to respond appropriately to various stimuli, you may be able to "switch off" your asthma. We have seen children who have learned these techniques by trial and error. The usefulness of breathing exercises lies in learning to relax and not panic while waiting for medication to work. Individualized behavior modification can be integrated into the treatment of your asthma.

Can My Job Make My Asthma Worse?

Obviously yes, if your environment exposes you to substances to which you are allergic. Some examples are the following:

• Animals — guinea pigs, rabbits, and mice (laboratory workers)

- Pollen (gardeners)
- Dust and molds (housekeepers and janitors)
- Fish (food handlers)

Nonallergic irritating substances may also cause asthma.

- Exhaust fumes (auto mechanics)
- Chemical substances (factory workers)
- Sawdust (carpenters)
- Cigarette smoke (bartenders)

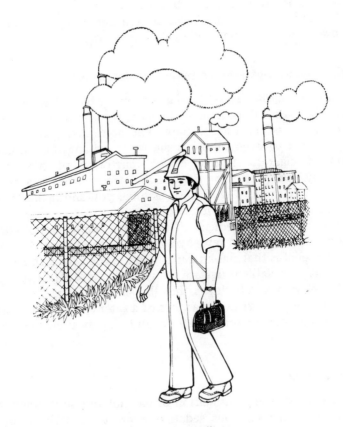

Occupational allergy.

If you notice relief from asthma on your days off, you should suspect that the cause of your asthma may be work related. Quitting your job may not always be a desirable solution. If this is the case, taking certain asthma medicines before going to work and wearing a face mask may help. You should encourage your employer to improve ventilation or, if possible, transfer you to another work location where you will not be exposed to the troublesome substance.

Can Asthma Be Caused by Allergy to Tobacco Smoke?

Yes. This has been documented with positive skin tests and special blood tests. It is rare but may occur at any age.

Usually, tobacco smoke is a nonallergic irritant which causes more irritation in allergic individuals.

What About Cigarette Smoking and Marijuana?

Tobacco smoke is a strong irritant which triggers the bronchospasm of asthma. Asthmatics who smoke often deny the adverse effects of their habit; yet, nonsmoking asthmatics report that tobacco smoke is the worst irritant of all. Inhalation of cigarette smoke causes narrowing of the small bronchial tubes and counteracts the effects of asthma medications. In short, if you have asthma, you and members of your household should not smoke.

The "active" ingredient of marijuana smoke, tetrahydrocannabinol (THC), is actually a mild bronchodilator. A popular misbelief is that smoking marijuana is good for asthmatics. Currently available drugs are many times more effective than THC. New research shows that the smoke of one "joint" is twenty times as irritating as that of a filter cigarette! Regular use of marijuana worsens asthma and may even cause COPD or emphysema.

Can I Drink Alcohol?

Yes. Whereas the combination of alcohol and antihistamines can act as a dangerous sedative, there is no such harmful interaction between alcohol and bronchodilators such as theophylline, metaproterenol, terbutaline, and adrenalin. Moderate amounts of alcohol are not known to have any effect on asthma.

You might be allergic to certain ingredients of alcoholic beverages. If you wheeze after drinking wine, for example, you can select other types of alcoholic beverages to help identify the responsible ingredient.

Sex?

Some asthmatics are greatly disturbed by the wheezing which often accompanies lovemaking. Actually, this is frequently the same as exercise-induced wheezing and may simply be an exacerbation of previously ignored mild asthma. Proper medication can usually control the wheezing. Sometimes a spray or bronchodilator before sex is all that is necessary.

Should I Get Pregnant?

Most asthmatics go though pregnancy and delivery without complications but extreme cases may compromise the health of the fetus. Complex hormonal changes occur during pregnancy, and these can make your asthma better or worse. You may need to modify your asthma medications during this period.

Can I Take Asthma Medications if I Am Pregnant?

You should continue taking medications under your physician's direction. The best medication is theophylline; there have been no reports of adverse effects to the unborn baby. Your physician may prescribe other medicines, such as terbutaline, metaproterenol, cromolyn, and inhaled steroids, such as Vanceril, which all have been safely used during pregnancy. If your symptoms are severe, moderate doses of prednisone may be required. In addition, severe attacks may be treated with adrenalin. Asthma-related drugs that should be avoided in pregnancy include the antihistamine brompheniramine

(Dimetapp, Dimemtane), hydroxyzine (Atarax, Marax, Vistaril), phenergan and iodides (cough preparations), and tetracyclines.

Is Asthma Contagious?

Asthma itself is not contagious. Your closest friends are safe and cannot catch your asthma. If your asthma is accompanied by an infection such as influenza, however, you can spread the infection.

Can I Play Sports?

Would you like to win an Olympic medal? Sure you can! Some of the best athletes in the Olympic games have asthma! The days of being restricted from participating in sport activities are gone. With newer medicines and treatments for asthma, you stand an equal chance to come out a winner. The key to winning is control of your asthma by doing everything your physician tells you to do and taking the prescribed medicines before competing.

Exercise should be an essential part of the overall care of your asthma. If you can tolerate it, aerobic exercise is ideal. Aerobic exercise includes running, swimming, and energetic dancing; it improves the ability of muscles to use oxygen efficiently, thus increasing endurance. Many asthmatics tolerate swimming best. With less than optimal control you may have to settle for less strenuous activities such as bowling, golf, and light weight training.

What About Backpacking?

Backpacking may result in some excessive exposure to pollens at certain times of the year. If you are allergic to grass, don't backpack on a valley floor in April and May. However, immunotherapy with allergy shots can alleviate the problem. If the exertion of the backpacking triggers wheezing, then an appropriate bronchodilator or Intal should be used beforehand. You should not avoid this excellent physical outdoor activity, but severe asthmatics should *not* be isolated from emergency medical services.

What Is the Best Medicine for Asthma?

The best medicine for asthma is the bronchodilator theophylline, which is available in many commercial preparations by prescription (aminophylline, Slo-Phyllin, Theo-Dur). Theophylline may be taken alone or in combination with metaproterenol (Alupent) or terbutaline (Brethine) in order to relax the spasm of the smooth muscles of the bronchial tubes. Older preparations (Tedral and Marax) have a combination of drugs that may also be helpful.

Cromolyn sodium (Intal) is a relatively new medication that works by preventing the spasm of the bronchial tubes. It is useful for younger allergic patients, especially before exercising.

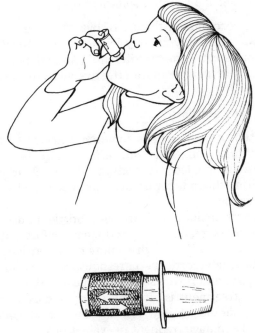

Inhalation of Intal by spinhaler.

Every Six Hours! Are You Kidding?

When asthma is mild and intermittent, occasional use of medication may be adequate. For the best relief of ongoing asthma, regular medication is necessary. Liquid and regular theophylline tablets must be taken every six hours around the clock in order to achieve full therapeutic levels in the blood. Newer timed-release capsules and tablets may be taken every eight to twelve hours, but they still must be taken on a regular basis because their onset of action is slow. The level of theophylline in the blood should be measured when your wheezing fails to clear with the usual dose as an increase may be necessary. Metaproterenol by mouth or inhalation and oral terbutaline may be used on an intermittent basis. Any cortisone should be taken exactly as prescribed and should be taken for a definite period of time, not "as needed."

Can I Use Over-the-Counter Asthma Sprays?

We do not recommend the use of over-the-counter medicines for asthma without your physician's advice. Newer inhalant preparations such as metaproterenol (Alupent) or isoetharine (Bronkometer) may be more effective and are longer acting.

Should I Take Steroids?

The addition of cortisone is sometimes necessary to control severe asthma. Dangerous side effects may be avoided by using the new inhaled preparations (Vanceril or Beclovent) or by limiting the number of days that you take high doses of oral prednisone.

Side effects include weight gain, brittle bones, diabetes, high blood pressure, cataracts, and menstrual irregularity. The most serious side effect is the failure of the adrenal glands to produce adequate cortisone in response to stress such as accidents, surgery, and future severe asthma attacks.

Cortisone treatment is often necessary and extremely beneficial. You should closely follow your physician's specific instructions and have frequent re-evaluations.

Which Drugs Must I Avoid if I Have Asthma?

Certain drugs can trigger an attack in asthmatic patients. These include propanolol (Inderal) which is sometimes used for heart conditions and high blood pressure and occasionally for migraine headaches and hyperthyroid disorders. These should always be avoided. Aspirin and other anti-inflammatory drugs such as Indocin, Butazolidin, Motrin, and rarely even Tylenol may be dangerous. Consult with your physician before taking these preparations or any new medications.

Should I Go to Asthma Camp?

There are several camps which provide educational and recreational programs for asthma patients. These programs deal with pertinent topics about asthma including its causes, prevention, and treatments. The participant is encouraged to enjoy the various recreational activities which also help to build self-esteem and confidence. While there are obvious advantages, not all are willing to participate because being at a special camp for asthmatics may reinforce the disheartening concept that having asthma places you in a category of "not normal" people; also, if your asthma is mild, you may find that such a camp is rather useless.

Whether you should go to an asthma camp is an individual decision. Ask your physician for advice.

Can I Die from Asthma?

Yes. Asthma can be fatal. Fortunately, proper use of new and improved medications has made death from asthma an uncommon occurrence. Early and prompt treatment minimizes the risk of fatal complications. You may need the intensive care available in a hospital. In spite of the potential mortality, asthmatics have a normal life expectancy.

When Shall I Call My Physician?

You and your physician should establish an individualized home treatment plan. This generally includes medications, adequate fluids, rest, and eliminating harmful environmental factors. If your asthma persists, call your physician.

Immediately call your physician if any of the following occur:

	Respiratory Rate Above	Heart Rate Above	Other Symptoms
Children	35	140	Exhaustion, irritability, severe vomiting, poor skin color, chest retractions
Adults	30	120	Severe vomiting, poor skin color, chest pains

If your physician is not available, call the closest emergency medical facility.

Should I Move?

Moving to a different city and environment may be of benefit if there will be less air pollution. Moving to avoid heavy pollen areas is not advisable. After a few seasons you are likely to develop new pollen allergies. Mold allergy patients often benefit from relocating to a drier climate.

Some allergens are unique and more prevalent in certain regions. Allergy specialialists can help to identify and treat the potential problem you might encounter.

Can Asthma Be Cured?

Asthma can be controlled. Bronchial tubes often remain irritable even after symptoms subside. Therefore, the disease may persist and always require attention. When the cat is removed, wheezing stops — but the asthma remains.

4

Skin Allergy

What Are Hives?

"Hives" is the common word for the condition *urticaria*, which is characterized by itchy "bumps" in the skin. They vary from pinhead size to welts several inches across. The hive (or *wheal*) is raised and pale and is usually surrounded by an area of redness and warmth (*erythema*).

Normal skin is peppered with mast cells, which contain histamine. The allergic reaction releases histamine into the skin, irritating nerve endings and thus causing itching. Histamine also causes tiny blood vessels in the skin to dilate and ooze clear serum. The serum in the skin results in the wheal, and the dilated blood vessels cause the erythema and warmth.

What Causes Hives?

Urticaria has many causes. Searching for the cause of urticaria is frustrating detective work for the patient and the allergist. Unfortunately, in most cases, the cause may never be found. Known causes of urticaria include

- Drugs
- Insect stings
- Foods
- Food additives
- Infections
- Parasites
- Colds
- Exercise
- Lupus erythematosus
- Cancer (rarely)

What Medications Cause Hives?

The list is extensive, including most, if not all, medications; the prime offenders are penicillin and aspirin. Sulfa drugs and some diuretics are frequent sensitizers. Codeine and barbiturates (phenobarbital) are on the list. The medication may have been recently started or may not have been used for many years. Repeated courses of therapy make sensitization and urticaria more likely.

Is Diet Important?

Food allergy is one of the most frequent causes of urticaria. Multiple foods have caused hives although each patient is usually allergic to only one or two. The list includes seafood, nuts, chocolate, strawberries, and other fresh fruits. Dairy products may also be responsible.

Food additives are prime suspects. In many cases, coal-tar-derived compounds, such as FD&C yellow dye No. 5 — tartrazine yellow — might be responsible. This additive is ubiquitous in our diet, especially in orange-flavored foods. It is used to make foods appear to be rich in eggs and is used to color some butter and margarine. Fresh oranges have been injected with tartrazine to improve their color! Some preservatives such as the benzoates (BHT and BHA) can cause urticaria. Trace amounts of antibiotics in food may also be responsible. This has occurred when patients who are sensitive to pencillin drink milk from penicillin-treated cows. Prepared foods may contain "hidden" ingredients such as nuts and eggs.

Are Hives Seasonal?

Occasionally, hives are caused by exposure to pollens and may recur each spring or fall. Rolling on grass may result in hives. Bringing pets into the house may cause urticaria in the winter. We have seen urticaria caused by allergy to mites and dog mange.

Are Hives Caused by Nerves?

Hives are frequently blamed on nerves. As in many illnesses, it is easy to say it is "nerves" when the real physical cause is unknown or difficult to find. Not all "nervous" people have hives but patients tell us that their hives are worse when they are nervous. Indeed, emotional upset or trauma can result in a flare of hives, but the development of urticaria does not necessarily mean you need counseling.

Can the Sun Cause Hives?

Yes. Physical factors such as the energy of sunlight can cause urticaria. Avoidance of sunlight and the use of sun screens such as A-Fil and Maxafil can prevent hives. No cure is known.

Exposure to cold temperatures may result in urticaria. This condition may be inherited. The medication Periactin is considered the best prevention for cold urticaria.

Can I Jog and Take a Sauna?

Physical activity and stress precipitate attacks; any exercise may exacerbate urticaria. Sauna baths and hot tubs may be intolerable.

One type of urticaria is specifically caused by heat and exercise. This is known as *cholinergic urticaria*. Atarax is the drug of choice.

Are Hives Dangerous?

Hives are not dangerous in themselves. Hives may be a warning of a more serious generalized anaphylactic reaction. Urticaria is sometimes associated with swelling of the lips, tongue, and throat. This conditions is known as *angioedema*. Angioedema of the larynx (voice box) constitutes a medical emergency requiring adrenalin and tracheotomy. In the case of cold urticaria jumping into cold water or drinking a cold liquid may cause a reaction.

Hereditary angioedema is a rare, frequently fatal disease involving swelling of the face, larynx, intestines, and extremities. The swelling does not itch but is very painful. Fortunately, new blood tests can easily provide the diagnosis of this condition, and the condition can be controlled by very small doses of synthetic hormones related to the male hormone *testosterone*. Acute attacks can be treated by transfusing the deficient serum proteins, but this treatment is new and expensive and available in only a few medical centers.

Are There Skin Tests for Hives?

In some cases, limited skin tests can determine an inhalant or food allergy. Skin tests can help diagnose penicillin allergy but are not useful with other drugs. Skin testing can diagnose allergy to bee stings, a cause of sudden urticaria.

A thorough medical history remains the best diagnostic tool. Elimination and medically supervised challenges of suspect substances remain the only true test.

Can Medication Cure Hives?

No. Medications are very helpful, however, in controlling the symptoms of urticaria. Antihistamines are the drug of choice; chlorpheniramine (Chlor-Trimeton), diphenhydramine (Benadryl), and hydroxyzine (Atarax) are commonly used. Specific recommendations include Periactin for cold urticaria and Atarax for cholinergic urticaria. Acute, severe attacks may be helped by adrenalin. Your physician may also try oral adrenalinlike drugs. Cortisone may be added for short-term control in severe cases.

What Is Eczema?

Eczema is a skin eruption that is itchy, red, and dry. This condition may be acute or chronic.

The chronic type of eczema that is observed in the early years of life is commonly called *atopic dermatitis* and frequently occurs in highly allergic patients. There are often well-defined allergic causes of the eczema itself, and these individuals frequently develop respiratory allergies, such as hayfever and asthma, later on.

The acute forms of eczema includes poison oak, skin infections, metal contact sensitivities, detergent irritations, and pityriasis rosea, a severe but transient rash of unknown cause.

Is Eczema Always Allergic?

No. Eczema can occur in response to exposures to a variety of nonallergic irritating substances such as detergents and industrial chemicals (irritant contact dermatitis). It can also be seen as a reaction to chronic scratching (neurodermatitis) and gets worse when one perspires heavily.

The allergy type of eczema results from exposure to an allergen with a specific immune response. Allergic eczema is divided into atopic dermatitis and contact dermatitis. Further discussion of eczema will be limited to atopic dermatitis.

Is Eczema Infectious?

The skin affected by eczema generally becomes infected very easily. The breakage of the skin that results from scratching itchy skin allows bacteria to enter. Signs of significant skin infection include increased weeping, crusting, and swelling.

Once the infection begins, it can spread from a localized area to a generalized skin infection.

The invading bacteria are "staph" (*Staphlococcus*) and occasionally "strep" (*Streptococcus*). These organisms must be eradicated with systemically administered antibiotics as soon as possible.

Good hygiene and control of your itching are critical in the prevention of serious skin infections.

What Parts of the Body Are Affected?

All parts of the body can be affected, but noticeable lesions tend to develop in those areas where the individual is most likely to reach and scratch.

During infancy, the cheeks and the skin behind the ears are affected first. Then, the eczema lesions may "spread" to the forehead and outer surfaces of the arms and legs. The folds of the elbows and knees, the ankles and wrists, and sides of the neck are classic sites for subsequent involvement.

Can I Be Vaccinated?

Smallpox vaccination is never allowed because of the severe and fatal complications that can occur in individuals with eczema. The vaccine contains live cowpox viruses which induce immunity to smallpox, and eczema patients have a deficient immunological status which allows the vaccine virus to proliferate and cause a serious life-threatening infection. Even if your eczema is under control, you still should not receive this vaccination. In fact, smallpox vaccinations are not suggested in the family of an eczema patient.

Other vaccinations such as the childhood immunization shots to pertussis (whooping cough), diphtheria, tetanus, mumps, measles, and rubella (German measles) are allowed.

Does Eczema Change With Age?

Eczema can begin and resolve spontaneously at any age. In most patients, eczema is apparent by the age of two years. It is often seen, however, in the first few weeks of life.

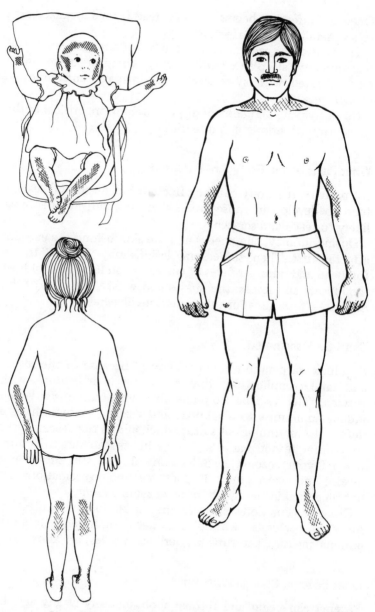

Sites of eczema on children (left) and adult (right).

Infantile eczema usually clears spontaneously. Some may continue to be afflicted throughout their childhood years. The sites of involvement change from the face to the arms and legs.

Childhood eczema often clears by puberty. Adult eczema can be present in various patterns, appearing most commonly on the hands.

Is Eczema Associated With Asthma?

There is a strong correlation between asthma and a history of childhood eczema. It has been reported that, based on retrospective studies, one-third of the eczema patients with a family history of allergies will develop asthma.

If your child has eczema, you may be able to prevent later serious allergies such as asthma. You should continue to avoid known food allergens. Do not ask for problems by bringing pets into your house, using feather pillows, and allowing your child to sleep in a dusty room.

Will My Eczema Get Worse in Cold Climate?

You can expect your eczema to worsen in a colder climate, especially at higher altitudes where the air contains less moisture, making your skin dry and itchy. At low temperatures, you might also be tempted to wear wool clothing which can further irritate the skin.

On the other hand, many patients find that their eczema completely clears when they go to tropical areas. Aloha!

Can My Dog Be the Cause of My Eczema?

Yes! And other pets can cause it, too. You might not observe any obvious association between dog exposure and worsening of your skin condition. However, if skin tests show that you are sensitive to dog allergen, you may only need to come in contact with dried dog saliva or small amounts of dander left in the living room to make your eczema flare. The same rule also applies to other animals such as cats, hamsters, mice, and horses.

Can Orange Juice Make My Eczema Worse?

Yes. Certain foods can make eczema worse for a particular patient. The food is not always the cause of the eczema; nevertheless, the allergic individual may often be specifically sensitive to foods in addition to a specific inhalant such as pollen, dust, or animal dander. The food in question may be oranges or other fruits, wheat, and so on. When properly carried out, trial elimination diets will identify the foods that make the eczema flare up. Again, skin testing may be of some help in diagnosis.

Why Do I Itch So Much?

Everybody feels a little itch most of the time. If you think about it, your skin itches in a few places right now; but this is usually ignored. Normal skin becomes more itchy with excessive dryness, especially with the frequent use of soaps in the winter.

If you have eczema, the itch is much more intense and your response to stimuli is exaggerated. Dry skin is the most important factor in eczema. The itchiness and dryness go hand in hand. Mechanical irritants such as wool and polyesters are major sources of difficulty for eczema patients.

Scratching is a normal response to itch, which may bring temporary relief. It does more harm than good. Scratching your dry, scaly skin will lead to infection and result in cracked, weeping lesions and subsequent scarring. This infected skin makes the itch become even more intense. Because of the altered state of immunity in eczema patients, skin infections are more common. Trimming fingernails, especially in eczema children, is advisable.

What Should I Wear?

Ideally nothing, but the best clothing is of loose-fitting cotton. This is the least irritating to the skin and allows better air circulation than tight-fitting noncotton garments. Avoid synthetic materials such as polyesters and nylons because they irritate the skin by allowing sweat and heat to accumulate. Also try to avoid rough fabrics such as wool.

Can I Go Sunbathing and Swimming?

Don't worry. Swimming is tolerated by those whose eczema is under good control. After swimming, skin lubricants should be immediately applied before the skin becomes excessively dry and itchy. Adequate chlorination and proper pH balance are essential. Salt water may cause a burning sensation and irritate your eczema skin.

What Soap Should I Use?

Ordinary soaps must be avoided because they are alkaline and remove the natural oils from the skin. Dove, Neutrogena, and Lowila are commonly recommended for the dry, itchy skin of eczema.

Cetaphil Lotion may serve as a cleanser for the skin and even as a shampoo.

Which Creams Are Best for Eczema?

It is important to keep your skin moist. This is best accomplished with the application of creams such as Eucerin and lotions such as Cetaphil. These should be applied at least twice a day; sometimes more frequent treatment is necessary.

Creams that contain urea, such as Carmol, soften the skin. They are often very helpful and may be used frequently, but you should not use such preparations on cracked and open eczema.

Cortisone creams and ointments are helpful. Hydrocortisone cream (1/2%) is available without a prescription. Stronger concentrations in a large variety of prescription preparations are often required. You should only use the weaker steroids on your face, groin, and underarms.

Tar compounds have been used for centuries — since King Tut's time — for relief of skin irritation. Tar and cortisone can be prescribed in combination to relieve itching as well as to soften and to moisturize.

Will Vaseline Help?

Vaseline should *not* be used. It will coat the skin and seemingly soften it, but its occlusive nature (that is, it does not allow air to contact the skin) often contributes to a subsequent flare-up of the eczema.

Is Cortisone Really Necessary?

Yes, absolutely! It is important to remember that before cortisone was available, most eczema never came under good control. If used with proper caution, this medicine is effective and without side effects. In severe cases cortisone must be administered orally.

What Are the White Spots on My Child's Face?

These usually small areas of depigmentation on the face or extremities are called *pityriasis alba*. These spots represent the mildest form of eczema. They are more apparent during summer months with sun tans and in black children and can be successfully treated by using 0.5 percent hydrocortisone topically.

Should I Have Skin Tests?

Yes. Skin testing can detect those allergens which contribute to your eczema condition. The skin tests are particularly helpful for detecting inhalant or airborne allergens.

Will Allergy Shots Help My Eczema?

Infrequently, allergy shots will help. If your eczema is made worse during the pollen season, immunotherapy may be considered. Usually, this type of eczema is associated with pollen-induced hayfever or asthma. Allergy shots may make eczema worse and the dose may have to be reduced. In some cases, the shots may have to be discontinued.

When you are being treated with immunotherapy primarily for perennial respiratory allergies, you may initially experience a brief flare-up of your eczema. This does not usually interfere with treatment.

Are Poison Oak and Poison Ivy the Same?

Poison oak and poison ivy dermatitis occur primarily in North America; both give the same rash. The poison oak plant is found only in the West, however, while poison ivy grows in the East. They both produce oily *urushiols*, the oleoresins that sensitize the skin upon contact. Poison sumac is in the same category.

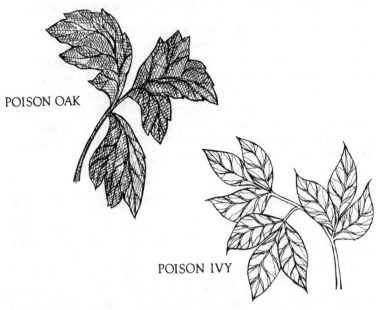

POISON OAK

POISON IVY

Poison oak and poison ivy.

Can I Get Poison Oak or Ivy From Clothing?

Yes. The oily resin will remain attached to articles of clothing until they are washed or dry cleaned. This contact, even months later, may result in a rash.

The same thing occurs when a pet has come into contact with the plant and then carries the resin home to a loving and affectionate family.

Can I Catch Poison Oak From Toilet Seats?

When President Nixon and his group visited China, the toilet seats had been newly lacquered in preparation for the visiting Americans. The lacquer contained a substance very similar to the allergen of poison oak. The native Chinese were not sensitive to this substance, but many of the Americans were. The bottom line, a very embarrassing situation for all concerned.

Do Allergic People Tend to Get Poison Oak or Ivy Easier?

Not really. In fact, there is evidence that patients with severe allergic eczema usually cannot become sensitized.

Poison oak/ivy is a different kind of allergy from hayfever, asthma, and associated eczemas. They cause a reaction which occurs in people who have sensitized white blood cells (T lymphocytes). The same type of delayed reaction is seen in allergic skin rashes from jewelry made with the most allergenic metal known, nickel. There are no special allergic antibodies of the IgE class in this kind of allergy.

How Can I Recognize the Rash of Poison Oak and Poison Ivy?

Poison oak and ivy start to break out one or two days after contact with the plant. This is termed a *delayed allergic reaction.*

The rash is initially red and slightly raised with small "bumps," which then enlarge and become filled with a clear watery fluid. Next, the rash begins to weep and ooze. A yellowish crust is formed and soon falls off leaving a very tender and sensitive layer of new skin exposed.

The face, arms, hands, and genital areas are the most commonly involved sites. Severe swelling often occurs in these sensitive tissues, especially the eyelids. The rash will often trace a "streaked" pattern which was brushed by the plant. As the rash progresses, this pattern is not as obvious.

There are degrees of severity. All the skin that is affected is extremely itchy and uncomfortable! The poison oak or ivy rash may last up to three to four weeks without cortisone therapy.

Will My Poison Oak or Poison Ivy Spread?

Infrequently, there will be systemic spread of the rash. This does not result from touching the rash and thereby externally transmitting it to another part of the body. The resin is no longer present when the rash has broken out. Instead, there is actually vascular (blood-borne) transmission so that the rash starts to appear at other sites.

Why Does the Rash Appear in Areas Where I Scratch? Am I Spreading It?

Yes, you can definitely "spread" the resin shortly after contact with the plant. The oily resin remains on the fingers and under the fingernails until it is washed off or removed. Therefore, it can make contact with other parts of the body which have not actually touched the plant.

You cannot spread the rash by touching it or scratching it after it has broken out. By this time, the resin is no longer present.

How Long Will It Last?

Poison oak and ivy last about two weeks. It is important to remember that if you are taking oral cortisone (prednisone), the treatment should last at least ten days.

What Is the Best Treatment for My Poison Oak or Ivy?

The best treatment is cortisone. If the rash is small and not too bothersome, the cortisone may be administered as a cream or spray. If the rash is severe or involves the eyelids or genitals, however, oral prednisone is usually necessary. This should be continued for at least ten days to provide control over the entire course of this malady. If the prednisone is stopped earlier, there is often a severe flare-up.

Antihistamines, such as Benadryl or Atarax, may be taken orally to help control the itching.

Should I Wash Off After Hiking to Remove the Resin Before the Rash Breaks Out?

No. Depending on your sensitivity, you only have from five minutes to an hour to possibly remove the oleoresin from your skin. Any washing should be done only with plain water; if you use a soap such as Fels Naptha or any reagent which "cuts grease," you may actually spread the remaining oily substance to other parts of your body.

Can You Get Poison Oak or Poison Ivy at High Altitudes?

No. They do not usually grow above 5000 feet.

Can Poison Oak and Poison Ivy Be Prevented?

An orally administered liquid preparation of the resin is available. The resin extract is taken daily in increasing doses before the season when poison oak and ivy flourish. This treatment is most important for persons who work outdoors in areas with heavy plant concentration, for example, telephone and electric line workers; it is only sometimes helpful, however, and research continues to develop more effective extracts.

Allergy shots for poison oak and poison ivy were used in the past. These caused many complications and are not recommended.

The American Indians used to give their babies poison oak leaves to chew in an effort to prevent later sensitivity. Do not attempt this.

5

Food Allergy

How Common Is Food Allergy?

Food allergy occurs in about 15 percent of adults and 40 percent of children who have other allergy symptoms. In infancy, allergy almost always includes food sensitivity.

How Does Eating Foods Cause Allergy?

Ingestion of foods can cause allergy in several ways. Symptoms may be immediate or delayed by many hours. The immediate reactions are the result of sensitization and production of IgE antibodies, similar to the sensitization process in hayfever. Briefly, exposure to specific food proteins causes the formation of IgE allergy antibodies. These antibodies attach to mast cells in the skin and in the digestive and respiratory systems. When the food is eaten again, the protein combines with IgE and histamine is released. The reaction may vary greatly in severity from mouth itching to generalized anaphylaxis and shock. Common symptoms include hives, angioedema, wheezing, vomiting, cramps, and diarrhea. Nasal symptoms may also be present. Almost any food can be responsible. Common sensitizers include seafoods, nuts, fresh fruits, eggs, and legumes.

Delayed onset reactions include allergic rhinitis or hayfever, wheezing, headache, and abdominal pain. Delayed food allergy is more common in children. This reaction is not due to IgE antibodies and involves other immune mechanisms. Foods eaten on a regular basis, such as dairy foods, wheat products, and corn products, are more likely to be responsible.

Which Are the Most Common Allergenic Foods?

It is no wonder that cow's milk is the most common, since this is the food that most of us feed our newborn infants. Its products—cheese, yogurt, butter—are major food items in our diets. It is also present as the milk solids in popular commercially baked products, such as breads and cookies.

Egg is another common food allergen, especially the egg white. Egg whites contain a highly allergenic protein called *albumin*. This protein is often found in pastries and breads. Only rarely will an egg-sensitive individual also be allergic to chicken.

Of the cereal grains, the most common offenders are wheat and corn. These should be introduced slowly and only after rice and oats have been tolerated.

Legumes, for example, peanuts, are often associated with immediate allergic reactions. Soybeans, another legume, are also allergenic and are growing in popularity in our diets. More soybean allergies are expected in the near future. Did you know that licorice is also a legume?

Seafoods, especially shellfish, are notoriously well known for their severe immediate allergic reactions. A sensitive individual can actually experience an asthma attack simply by smelling the odor of fish or shellfish.

Chocolate often causes headaches and skin rashes. Cola drinks and cocoa containing foods should also be avoided in chocolate-sensitive individuals.

What Is the Best Way to Diagnose Food Allergy?

The most reliable method of diagnosing food allergy is the trial elimination diet. If a limited number of selected foods are properly eliminated for two to three weeks, the allergen is most often identified. The return of the symptoms after subsequent challenges may help to confirm the diagnosis. However, most patients are not too anxious to make themselves sick again after achieving a significant remission. Such challenges are really only necessary when the improvement is not clear cut and remains questionable. A subsequent challenge is not to be carried out when the reaction is life threatening.

If you would like to uncover a possible allergy to milk, wheat, corn, and legumes the following diets will be helpful. Ideally, only one food should be tested at a time. On rare occasions, the basic elimination diet (pg. 64) is necessary and can be very helpful. Chocolate and cola beverages should always be avoided when food allergies are being investigated because they are frequent offenders.

Remember, any cheating or mistakes will invalidate the test diet. Keep a careful record of symptoms prior to and during the trial period. A current illness, such as a respiratory infection, will, of course, interfere with the test.

Are Skin Tests Helpful?

Skin tests for foods by the scratch method may provide some help with diagnosis. They can be misleading for delayed-onset reactions and must be interpreted in the light of clinical history: the age of onset of symptoms, the types of foods in the diet, and, most important, the results of a trial elimination diet.

Skin tests are useful in the diagnosis of immediate reactions. Since systemic allergic reactions can occur from the testing itself, this procedure must be carefully undertaken after a thorough history. When a specific food is suspected as the cause of a severe reaction, we begin testing with diluted test material.

Routine skin testing for a large number of foods is rarely necessary or helpful. Be skeptical if testing of 30 or more foods is suggested.

Are There Blood Tests for Food Allergies?

Yes, but not for all types of allergic reactions. If the clinical reaction is immediate, the RAST blood test (pg. 12) will usually be reliably positive for the suspected food. If the reaction is delayed and results only after the food is eaten repeatedly, this test may be misleading.

In most cases the RAST test is not necessary for the diagnosis of food allergies. If your reaction was life threatening, then your physician may want to do the laboratory RAST before skin testing. Additionally, a positive RAST may sometimes confirm a suspect food allergen which gave a negative skin test.

When properly performed, RAST testing can provide important information. As with skin testing, however, the results must be carefully interpreted in the light of the patient's clinical history.

Have Specific Allergens Been Identified for Food Alergies?

Yes, but only for a limited number of foods. The milk protein allergens are casein, alpha lactalbumin, beta lactoglobulin, and bovine serum albumin. When milk is separated into curds and whey, the curd becomes cheese and the predominant protein is casein; whey is an odoriferous liquid containing the other three allergenic proteins. Whey is commonly used in food processing, especially in bakery goods. Casein is also present in goat's milk, so this is not always an adequate substitute.

The protein complex DS-22 has been identified as the allergen in cod fish.

A glycoprotein is thought to be the allergenic substance common to legumes: peas, beans, soybean, peanuts, and licorice.

Are Food Allergy Shots Helpful? How About Sublingual Drops?

Food allergy shots and sublingual drops have not been demonstrated to be helpful when controlled studies are carried out. While patient testimonies exist to suggest the efficacy of food shots and even food drops placed under the tongue, these forms of treatment remain controversial.

The only reliable treatment for food allergy is elimination.

Is My Asthma Caused by Food Allergy?

Asthma with severe wheezing and intermittent coughing with bronchospasm may indeed be caused by food allergy. Even asthma that is only present with physical exertion may improve with a trial elimination diet.

Before you start such a diet, your allergy specialist will take a thorough history with your physical examination. Necessary studies include a chest X-ray, breathing tests for pulmonary function, and skin testing. Other tests that may be indicated are sinus X-rays, a sweat test, blood tests, sputum studies for infections and eosinophils, and an electrocardiogram (ECG).

Above all, remember: not all that wheezes is asthma — and not all asthma is allergy.

Can Food Allergy Cause Hayfever Symptoms?

Yes. The symptoms of food allergy with nasal congestion and discharge together with sneezing can result from food allergies.

If you are allergic to foods as well as pollens, you may be exquisitely sensitive to even small amounts of food during the pollen season. Your specific food elimination must be very strict without any "slip-ups." At other times of the year, a less rigid diet may be tolerated and perennial symptoms will usually remain under adequate control.

Indeed, with trial elimination diets and subsequent challenges, foods have been clearly demonstrated to be the cause of typical respiratory allergic symptoms.

Does Alcohol Increase the Risk of a Severe Allergic Immediate Reaction to Foods?

Yes. When you are at a party and have a few drinks, you will be relaxed and not concentrating on what is on the hors d'oeuvres tray. If you are sensitive to certain nuts or sesame seeds, this is the most frequent "set-up" for a severe, life-threatening allergic reaction to those nuts or the sesame seeds which may be part of the snacks. Also, some allergists have felt that alcohol facilitates rapid absorption of food allergens, accelerating the allergic reaction. Beware! You cannot let your guard down.

Which Foods Should Be Avoided During Infancy?

Exclusive breast feeding for the first six months is the best food, especially for the allergy-prone infant. If this is not possible, a soybean formula substitute or Nutramigen should be tried. Soy occasionally causes allergies and may need to be avoided if sensitivity develops.

The most allergic foods are cow's milk, eggs, wheat, corn, and the legumes—peas, beans, and soybeans; these should be avoided for the first year. In addition, if there is a strong family history of allergic reactions to other foods, these foods should also be excluded from the diet.

What Foods Should I Introduce First in My Baby?

Breast milk is nutritious and is the recommended food for infants. Iron, fluoride and vitamins A, C, and D are the only supplements that may be necessary for complete nutrition in the breast-fed baby for the first year of life. Thereafter, the introduction of selected foods should be gradual. Each new food should be added to the diet at two-week intervals so that if any adverse food reaction occurs, that food can be easily identified and removed from the diet.

For the allergy-prone infant, breast milk should be continued as long as possible. Soy milk may be introduced cautiously at six months, and cow's milk after one year of age. Solid foods should be delayed for at least six months; then begin with cereals. As for cereals, rice and oats are the least allergenic and should be introduced before wheat and corn. Eggs should not be added until after the age of one year.

Should I Breast Feed?

Yes. The best food for the normal newborn baby is breast milk. Although commercially prepared milk formulas are easily available and often are more convenient to feed, breast milk is superior. It is not allergenic, has higher bioavailability for zinc, iron, and other minerals, and is far more economical.

Breast milk provides the major advantage of immunologic protection against food allergies and invading infectious organisms. It contains naturally occurring IgA antibodies which protect the infant's immature gastrointestinal system. Commercial formulas do not contain these protective IgA antibodies.

Doesn't Everybody Need Milk?

"One man's food is another man's poison." This old saying is especially true about milk. Most conventional milk formulas are cow's milk. Many infants become sick by developing either allergy or intolerance to it.

Milk proteins can easily sensitize the allergy-prone infant, and, once sensitized, the infant may develop eczema, congestion, coughing, and diarrhea. The child can become seriously ill and hospitalization sometimes may be necessary.

Milk intolerance is even more common. This occurs as a result of an enzymatic deficiency in the intestines. The enzyme *lactase* is necessary to metabolize the lactose sugar which is present in cow's milk. Those who are deficient in this enzyme would experience vomiting, bloating, cramps, and diarrhea after milk ingestion. Among Asians and blacks, percent have lactase deficiency by the time they reach adulthood. When powder milk was sent to underdeveloped countries, the black population used it for wall paint, recognizing that milk invariably would induce diarrhea when they drink it.

When the problem is caused by cow's milk during infancy, the milk is often replaced by a soy formula, but sensitization to soy may also occur. Other types of milk (goat's milk or Nutramigen) may have to be tried. As the infant's diet expands to include solids, milk becomes less important as a food source.

You can totally eliminate milk from the diet once your child begins to eat adequate amounts of meat and vegetables; however, calcium and vitamin D may not always be adequately supplied in the diet of a non-milk-drinking child. You can obtain calcium with fortified vitamin D without a prescription. And whenever making homemade soups, throw the bones in!

Can You Suggest Any Food Substitutes?

1. Cow's milk: Soy is the most frequently used substitute. Beware, however; the glycoprotein of soybean also may be allergenic.

2. Corn and wheat: Various grains, such as rice, barley, and rye, may be substituted for corn and wheat. Read labels carefully since few breads are made without wheat.

3. Chocolate: Carob is a good substitute for chocolate but, again, remember that carob is a legume related to peas, beans, and soybeans.

4. Citrus: Other fruit juices and nectars may be adequate substitutes with the reminder that most nectars contain 25 percent corn syrup which need not necessarily be mentioned on the label.

5. Nuts: These are often found in minute quantities in bakery products such as cookies. An extremely sensitive person should not trust any commercial cookies even if the label does not mention nuts. You can only be sure about the cookies you bake on your own.

6. Fish: It is not difficult to substitute meat for fish. However, severe life-threatening reactions have occurred when patients who are allergic to fish are exposed to the odors of this food. Beware of walking into a house or restaurant where fish is being cooked.

It is wise to use a substitute sparingly; otherwise, you may develop sensitivity to the new food. Don't jump from the frying pain into the fire.

Elimination diets for some of the more allergenic foods can be found on pages 65–68.

How About Poi as a Milk Substitute?

In the South Seas, poi is used as a milk substitute. Derived from the taro root, it provides a hardy food substance with minimal allergic potentials.

Is Colitis an Allergy?

Colitis often improves with the elimination of certain foods. The first food you should eliminate for a trial period is milk; this gives the best and the most frequent results. Certain drugs, such as ampicillin, may also cause colitis. Gluten-containing grains, such as wheat, may affect the small intestine and result in a serious problem called *celiac disease*. In some, this may well be an allergic disease, although the immunological mechanisms have not yet been demonstrated.

Basic Elimination Diet

FOODS ELIMINATED

Milk
Chocolate and cola
  beverages
Egg
Citrus fruits (orange,
  lemon, grapefruit)
Legumes
Tomato
Corn

Wheat
Rice
Oats
Barley
Rye
Millet
Food colors and preserva-
  tives
Cinnamon

O.K. TO USE

Apple, apple juice, apple-
  sauce
Banana, pear
Grape, grape juice, vinegar,
  raisin
Pineapple, pineapple juice
Almond, apricot, cherry,
  peach, plum, prune
Cranberry, blueberry,
  raspberry, blackberry,
Loganberry, strawberry,
  gooseberry
Fig
Persimmon
Rhubarb, buckwheat
Coconut, date
Papaya
Vanilla
Ginger, arrowroot

Clove
Mint
Tea
Hazel nut, wintergreen
Cashew nut
Brazil nut
Pine nut
Olive
Avocado
Cucumber, pickles, squash,
  pumpkin, cantaloupe,
  melons
Mushroom
Sweet potato
Radish, turnip, broccoli,
  cabbage, brussels sprouts,
  Chinese cabbage, collards,
  kale
Carrot, celery

Artichoke, lettuce
Beet, spinach, swiss chard
Cauliflower
Asparagus, onion
Green pepper, red pepper
Sugar (maple, brown, white)

Clams, abalone, scallops,
   oysters, shrimp, lobster
Fish
Chicken, turkey, lamb

Milk Elimination Diet

FOODS ELIMINATED

- Liquid milk or cream, whether used as a drink, on cereal, on fruit, or elsewhere
- Evaporated milk, dried milk, skimmed milk,* goat's milk
- Cottage cheese and all other cheeses; yogurt, custard, junket
- Ice cream and sherbet (sherbet contains as much milk protein as ice cream)
- Pancakes and waffles made with milk (many mixes contain dried milk and should not be used)

O.K. TO USE

- All foods that are not specifically eliminated above may be eaten; all meats, vegetables, and fruits are allowed.
- The following foods have traces of milk solids, but are allowed in the diet: bakery products including bread, rolls, cookies, cakes and pies; butter and margarine.†
- Mocha Mix and Coffee Rich are cream substitutes; use them on cereals and for cooking (pancakes and waffles); they may be too rich to be used as a drink, but some drink them after adding water.

*Skimmed milk is lower in fat but contains, relative to calories, a large amount of the allergenic protein.
†Patients with extreme sensitivity will react to these traces of milk. These patients are unusually aware of their milk because of the severe symptoms that follow milk ingestion.

- Soybean milks can be substituted for cow's milk in infants; Nutramigen and Gerber's meat base are also good substitutes.

If milk elimination is to be continued after this trial diet, a calcium substitute may be used in children.

Corn Elimination Diet

Some of the following foods need not be eliminated entirely. Exceptions and substitutes are listed under "O.K. to Use" for those items marked with an asterisk (*).

FOODS ELIMINATED

Corn syrup

Canned fruits and nectars   Jams and jellies*
Peanut butter*   Ice cream*
Mayonnaise*   Catsup
Sweetened cereals   Pancake syrup*
Mocha-Mix and Coffee-Rich   Candies

Corn cereal

Fresh, canned, frozen corn   Hominy grits
Popcorn   Corn flakes
Fritos   Cheerios
Cornmeal   Beer
Mexican food

Corn starch

Chinese food (not all)   Prepared bakery products
Prepared gravies and soups   Powdered sugar

Corn meal and corn flour

Corn bread   Pancake and waffle mixes
Corn muffins   Fish sticks

Corn oil

Mazola*   Margarine
Potato chips*   Salad oil and dressing

O.K. TO USE

Best Foods mayonnaise,   Olive oil
  Hellman's mayonnaise   Natural peanut butter
Brockmeyer's ice cream   Potato chips without corn
Homemade jams and jellies   oil
Pure maple syrup   Arrowroot (for thickening)
Spry, Crisco, Wesson Oil,

Wheat Elimination Diet

FOODS ELIMINATED

- Ordinary flour: in general, *all* regular bakery goods
- Bread: crackers, buns, biscuits, graham crackers, wafers, pancakes, cones, wheat matzos, macaroons, cakes, cookies, dumplings, doughnuts, pretzels, pie crust, rolls, wheat germ, many cereals
- Pasta and noodles: macaroni, spaghetti, vermicelli, ravioli
- Foods with cereal or bread fillers: stuffing, gravy, chili, cream sauces, meatloaf, fried food coatings
- Postum

O.K. TO USE

- Ry-Krisp
- Rice Krispies
- Cream of Rice
- Oatmeal
- Tapioca and arrowroot
- Potato, rice, and soy flour
- Grainless mix

Wheat- and gluten-free products can be purchased at reliable health food stores.

Legume Elimination Diet

FOODS ELIMINATED

- Beans
- Peas
- Soybean
- Peanuts

- Licorice
- Tragacanth
  (vegetable gum)
- Alfalfa

Recipes to Send for

Wheat, Milk and Egg-Free Recipes (free)
  Quaker Oats Company
  Consumer Service
  Merchandise Mart Plaza
  Chicago, Illinois 60654
125 Great Recipes for Allergy Diets (75 cents)
  Good Housekeeping
  Bulletin Service
  Box 2317
  FDR Station
  New York, New York 10150
Allergy Recipes (wheat, milk and egg free) ($1.50)
  The American Dietetic Association
  Publication BO305
  430 North Michigan Avenue
  Chicago, Illinois 60611
Diets Unlimited for Limited Diets ($5.00)
  Allergy Information Association
  Room 7
  25 Poynter Drive
  Weston, Ontario M9R1K8
  CANADA
Isomil Cookbook for Infants (milk free) (free)
  Ross Laboratories
  Department 441
  625 Cleveland Avenue
  Columbus, Ohio 43216

Soyalac (milk free) (free)
  Loma Linda Foods
  Medical Products Division
  Riverside, California 92505
The Milk-Free Cookbook for Infants (free)
  Syntex Laboratories Inc.
  Nutritional Products Division
  Palo Alto, California 94304

If I Have a Food Allergy, Will Other Foods in the Same Family Cause a Reaction?

Yes, especially if your reaction was severe and immediate. The following will serve as a guide.

FOOD PLANT FAMILIES

Family	Related Plants
Apple	Apple
	Loquat
	Pear
Banana	Chestnut
Birch	Filbert
	Hazelnut
Buckwheat	Dock
	Rhubarb
Cashew	Mango
	Pistachio
Citrus	Citron
	Grapefruit
	Kumquat
	Lemon
	Lime
	Orange
	Tangelo
	Tangerine
Cocoa	Coca leaf
	Chocolate
	Cola
	Karraya

Family	*Related Plants*
Ebony	Persimmon
Fungus	Morel
	Mushroom
	Truffle
Ginger	Turmeric
Goosefoot	Beet
	Lamb's quarters
	Spinach
	Swiss chard
Gourd	Cantaloupe
	Chinese watermelon
	Cucumber
	Gherkin
	Pumpkin
	Summer squash
	Watermelon
	Winter squash
Grape	American grape
	European grape
Grass	Bamboo
	Barley
	Canary grass
	Citronella
	Corn
	Millet
	Oats
	Popcorn
	Rice
	Rye
	Sorghum and milo
	Sugar cane
	Wheat
	Wild rice
Heather	Black huckleberry
	Blueberry
	Cranberry
Laurel	Avocado
	Bay leaf
	Cinnamon
	Sassafras

Family	Related Plants
Lily	Asparagus
	Chives
	Garlic
	Leek
	Onion
	Sarsaparilla
	Shallot
Madder	Black guava
	Coffee
Mallow	Cottonseed
	Durian
	Okra
Mimosa	Acacia
Mint	Basil
	Catnip
	Common mint
	Curled mint
	Lavender
	Marjoram
	Oregano
	Peppermint
	Sage
	Savory
	Spearmint
	Spike lavender
	Thyme
Morning glory	Sweet potato
Mulberry	Breadfruit
	Breadnut
	Fig
	Hop
Mustard	Broccoli
	Brussels sprouts
	Cabbage
	Chinese cabbage
	Collards and kale
	Garden cress
	Horseradish
	Kohlrabi

Family	*Related Plants*
	Radish
	Rape
	Rutabaga
	Sea kale
	Turnip
	Watercress
Myrtle	Allspice
	Chilian guava
	Clove
	Guava
Nasturtium	Bell pepper
	Cayenne pepper
	Chili
	Eggplant
	Potato
	Strawberry tomato
	Tomato
	Tree tomato
Nutmeg	Mace
Olive	Jasmine
	Manna
Orchid	Salep
	Vanilla
Palm	Cabbage palm
	Coconut
	Date
	Oil palm
Parsley	Anise
	Black cumin
	Caraway seed
	Carrot
	Celery and celeriac
	Coriander
	Cumin
	Dill
	Fennel
	Star anise
	Sweet cicily
	Sweet fennel
Passionflower	Passion fruit

Family	*Related Plants*
Pea (legumes)	Alfalfa
	Black-eyed pea, cowpea
	Carob bean
	Chick pea
	Clovers
	Common bean (navy, kidney, pinto, string)
	Jack bean
	Lentil
	Licorice
	Mesquite
	Peanut
	Soybean
	Tamarind
	Tragacanth
Pine	Juniper
	Pinyon nut
Plum	Almond
	Apricot
	Cherry
	Peach, nectarine
	Prune
	Sloe
	Wild cherry
Poppy	Poppyseed
Protea	Macadamia nut
Rose	Black raspberry
	Boysenberry, dewberry, loganberry
	Red raspberry
	Strawberry
Saxifrage	Currant
Senna	Tamarind
Spurge	Tapioca
Sunflower (aster)	Artichoke
	Camomile
	Chicory
	Dandelion
	Endive
	Jerusalem artichoke

Family	*Related Plants*
	Safflower
	Lettuce
	Sunflower seed
	Tarragon
Walnut	Butternut
	Hickory nut
	Pecan

OUTLINE OF ANIMAL FOODS

Amphibians	Frogs
Birds	Duck
	Goose
	Dove, squab
	Turkeys
	Guinea fowl
	Partridge and quail
	Chicken, guinea fowl, pheasant
Crustaceans	Crayfish
	Crabs
	Shrimp
	Lobsters
	Prawns
Fish	Sturgeon
	Smelts
	Eel
	Pompano
	Black bass, crappie, sunfish, herring, menhaden, sardine, shad, sprat
	Carp, chub
	Muskellunge, pickerel, pike
	Cod, haddock, pollack, whiting
	Hake
	Mullet
	Perch
	Flounder, halibut
	Grayling, red salmon, pink salmon, whitefish
	Croaker, drum, redfish, squeteague, weakfish

Family	Related Plants
	Bonito, mackerel, tuna
	Grouper, white bass, rock fish
	Bullhead, catfish
	Sole
	Porgy, red snapper
	Anchovy
	Swordfish
Mammals	Cow, goat, sheep
	Deer
	Hare, rabbit
	Squirrel
	Pig
Mollusks	Cockle
	Abalone
	Snail
	Periwinkle
	Clam
	Mussel
	Octopus
	Oyster
	Scallop
	Squid

6

Insect Allergy

How Do Insects Cause Allergy?

Some insects cause allergies by biting or stinging; others cause severe allergic reactions when their body parts or feces are inhaled. Bees, ants, fleas, and mosquitoes are part of the first group. The second group consists of house dust mites, cockroaches, crickets, caddis fly, and May fly.

Prevalence depends a great deal on geographic factors. The caddis and May flies are common severe problems in the Great Lakes region. Urban dwellers experience more cockroach allergy, whereas rural populations are more exposed to bees.

How About House Dust Mites?

One of the most important allergy components of house dust is the house dust mite, *Dermatophagoides*. This insect is 0.3 mm in length and barely visible without a microscope. With appropriate humidity and temperature during certain seasons, there is marked proliferation with an increased concentration of this insect. San Francisco and London provide favorable climates.

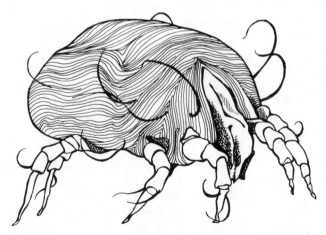

The house dust mite (magnified more than 200 times).

The house dust mite feeds on animal material with high protein content, especially human and animal dander; thus the name *Dermatophagoides*, "skin eater." It has been found and studied in Europe, America, and the Far East and is the allergen that makes house dust antigenically similar in these distant geographic locations.

Can I Be Allergic to Flea Bites?

Yes. Some patients develop large and extremely itchy local reactions to flea bites. In addition, some people are really bitten more than others. In areas where fleas are prevalent, repeated flea bites may actually desensitize you. Allergy shots may be considered for treating severe cases.

Will Vitamin B$_1$ (Thiamine) Help My Flea Bites?

Yes. An over-the-counter preparation, thiamine somehow elicits a noxious odor from the skin which repels fleas.

Where Is Cockroach Allergy a Problem?

New York City is probably the cockroach capital of the world! These insects are everywhere, however, and are extremely hardy. One cockroach can live on a drop of water for a year.

When they die or are exterminated, cockroaches are slowly pulverized and become a strong air-borne allergen. Their feces are also allergenic. Sensitized patients may develop asthma as well as nasal allergy symptoms.

What Are Fire Ants?

Fire ants (*Hymenoptera*) are close relatives of the bees and vespids (see pg. 81) and are found in the southern United States. They live in mounds in the ground. Fire ants first bite the victim with their jaws, then pivot their bodies, inflicting multiple stings. Both the bites and the stings are excruciatingly painful. Long-lasting local reactions with minute areas of dead skin may result. As with bees, the venom can cause severe, potentially fatal anaphylactic reactions. Immunotherapy is recommended in certain cases of sensitization.

How Is Insect Sting Allergy Diagnosed?

The most important diagnostic tool is a good history. If you are stung by an insect and develop hives on other areas of the body; or have other systemic signs or symptoms such as trouble breathing, generalized itching, or swelling of the tongue and throat; or go into anaphylactic shock — you have an allergy to that insect.

Skin testing with venom for the various insects will identify and confirm your specific sensitivity. Blood tests (RAST, see page 12) can also be done as part of the evaluation. The skin test is better than the blood test, since the RAST will not always pick up true bee sting sensitivity.

Will My Insect Allergy Reactions Become More Severe?

In most cases, subsequent insect stings will result in severe and even life-threatening reactions. Your immune system becomes more sensitive so that more IgE allergic antibodies are produced.

On the other hand, multiple stings will sometimes actually desensitize you with a mechanism similar to allergy shots. This can occur with allergic bee keepers; repeated stings, however, are potentially fatal.

Can Allergy to Insect Sting Be Cured?

Yes. You can receive allergy shots for bee sting and fire ant allergy as well as allergy to May fly and caddis fly. This treatment will desensitize you so that you will not react to subsequent stings. Ninety-five percent of patients who receive immunotherapy with bee venom are cured while they are receiving desensitizing injections.

If I Have Other Allergies, Should I Be Tested for Bee Stings?

No! Even though you may be more likely to develop a bee allergy than a nonatopic (nonallergic) individual, testing for bee sting allergy should only be done if allergic sensitivity is suspected because of a reaction following an actual bee sting. The testing itself may induce sensitivity, or even result in a life-threatening reaction; such tests should not be used to screen individuals simply because they have other allergies.

What Is Bee Venom?

Venom is a complex mixture of various chemicals. The main component of honeybee venom is a proteinlike substance called *mellitin*; mellitin causes pain and swelling after a sting. Other components are toxic to nerves. Phospholipase-A, an enzyme, is present in small amounts and is the component to which most people become allergic.

The venom of yellow jackets, wasps and hornets (vespids) contains no mellitin but does contain similar substances which cause even more intense pain. Honeybee venom and the venom of vespids also have components in common; thus, some persons who are sensitized to bees may later react to a sting of a hornet.

Bee venom is toxic. Even if you are not allergic to bee venom, it has been estimated that 500 simultaneous stings would be fatal.

If I Am Allergic to Yellow Jackets, Can I Also Be Sensitive to Honeybees?

Yes! Stinging insects such as the wasp, yellow jacket, hornet, and the honeybee share common allergenic components. These insects belong to the order *Hymenoptera*. Within this order, the wasp, hornet and yellow jacket all belong to the Vespid family.

The honeybee belongs to the Apid family and shares some allergens with the Vespids. If you are allergic to the yellow jacket, you are *most likely* to react to other vespids, but you can also be sensitive to the honeybee.

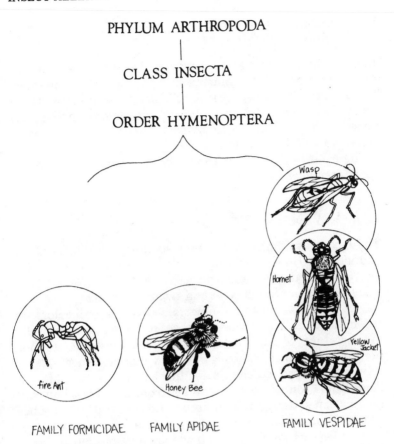

PHYLUM ARTHROPODA

CLASS INSECTA

ORDER HYMENOPTERA

Wasp

Hornet

Yellow Jacket

fire Ant

Honey Bee

FAMILY FORMICIDAE   FAMILY APIDAE   FAMILY VESPIDAE

Classification of stinging insects.

How Many People Die from Bee Stings?

In 2621 B.C., the first fatal reaction from a wasp or hornet sting was recorded in hieroglyphics on the walls of the tomb of the Egyptian king Menes. In the United States about 40 deaths occur each year from such insects as the hornet, wasp, and honeybee. For every death, however, there are thousands of severe and near-fatal reactions.

Who Should Be Given Shots for Bee Sting Allergies?

Immunotherapy should be reserved for those who have a definite history of systemic reaction to a bee sting, with positive results on tests specific for *Hymenoptera* venom. These reactions include difficulty breathing, fainting, and generalized hives. Progressive local reactions are warning signs of subsequent systemic reactions.

These high-risk patients should carry a medical emergency kit containing adrenalin.

How Can I Avoid Stings?

The key to avoiding stings is understanding the habits of bees and vespids. Honeybees will not fly when the temperature is less than 55 degrees and will also not fly on cloudy days. They are found around lakes and swimming pools.

Bees are attracted to red objects, so dark or drab colors are recommended. Wear long sleeves and avoid shorts. Walking barefoot is an invitation for trouble; so is wearing perfume. Of course, swatting at bees will provoke a sting.

In most urban communities, the keeping of bee hives is illegal. Bees journey for many miles from their hives and wild swarms can settle in trees or around houses. If possible, a bee keeper should remove any hive you may find. Remember, worker bees exposed to insecticide are irritable and are more likely to sting.

Wasps are found around houses, under eaves and behind gutters, hornets in trees and shrubs: their nests may be knocked down and burned. Similar to hornets, yellow jackets are, however, found in the ground. Yellow jackets are particularly likely to sting in the fall when the last, aggressive, hungry survivors of a colony are attracted to meat and garbage. They are found around picnic areas and around restaurant kitchens. Fast-acting pesticides may be helpful in local control of vespids; but consult a professional exterminator.

Should I Carry an Emergency Kit?

Positively! Life-threatening edema of the larynx (voice box), wheezing, and anaphylactic shock can occur within minutes. The sensitive person should carry adrenalin which can reverse the strangling edema and shock. The kits, whether commercially or personally set up, should contain injectable adrenalin and an oral preparation of antihistamines. The use of the adrenalin should be discussed with your physician; the dose will vary with age and weight, and great caution should be observed in patients with hypertension and heart disease. The adrenalin should be used only if systemic symptoms, such as respiratory distress, itching, or hives develop. The antihistamine should be taken after any sting. Antihistamines alone may cause drowsiness — be careful when driving.

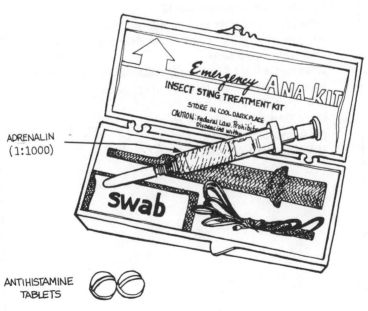

ADRENALIN
(1:1000)

ANTIHISTAMINE
TABLETS

Bee sting kit.

7

Allergy Shots

How Do Allergy Shots Work?

Immunotherapy alters your immune system in several ways. First, it stimulates the production of immunoglobulin G (IgG), another type of antibody which is specific for the allergen contained in the allergy extract. This antibody blocks the normally inhaled allergens from attaching to the sensitized mast cells. Consequently, the mast cells cannot release histamine and other mediators of the allergic response.

Second, immunotherapy makes the mast cells less responsive to allergenic stimuli. This is like hearing the ticking of a clock while trying to sleep. At first, the tick-tocks may keep you awake, but they become less irritating later as you adapt or become tolerant to the ticking noise. Likewise, the mast cells in your nose, eyes, and lungs become less reactive or more tolerant to the allergenic stimuli.

The third mechanism occurs when the body begins to produce suppressor lymphocyte cells that turn off the immune

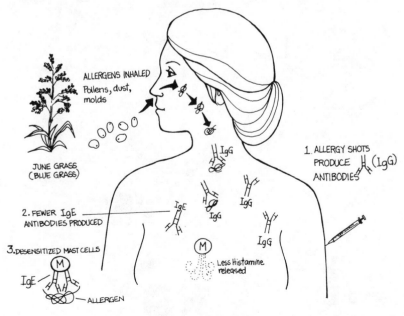

How allergy shots work.

system from producing harmful IgE antibodies. In this way, fewer IgE antibodies are available to attach to mast cells, thereby inhibiting a step for histamine release.

What Is the Allergy Shot?

The allergy shot contains an extract of the substance to which you are allergic. The extract is made by mixing specific allergens together with a special solution of salt water. Some extracts contain precipitated antigens for delayed absorption into the body tissues; these are useful for highly sensitive patients.

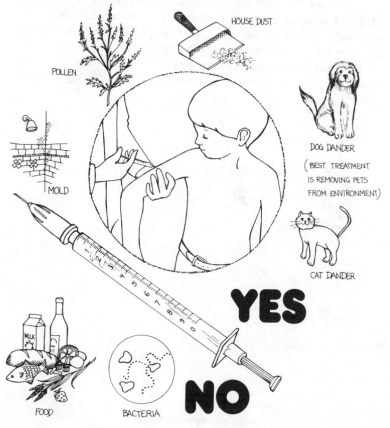

POLLEN

HOUSE DUST

MOLD

DOG DANDER

(BEST TREATMENT IS REMOVING PETS FROM ENVIRONMENT)

CAT DANDER

YES

FOOD

BACTERIA

NO

What allergy shots can (and cannot) do.

What Allergens Can Be Used?

Allergy antigen treatment should include inhalant allergens to which the patient is sensitive and which cannot be easily avoided. Pollens, dust, and mold allergens are the most commonly used. Animal danders may be used when significant symptoms occur and avoidance is impossible. Dander injections cannot be expected to help when a pet is in the house continually shedding dander. There is no good experimental evidence supporting the usefulness of food antigens and bacteria for allergy treatment.

When Should I Consider Taking Allergy Shots?

Immunotherapy with allergy shots should be considered when hayfever symptoms are severe enough to interfere with normal daily activities or when medications result in adverse reactions. Your job may not allow for the drowsiness caused by antihistamines; for example, you might fly an airplane or operate machinery. Blood pressure elevation may complicate the use of decongestants.

Treatment is also necessary when your allergy causes asthma with wheezing and persistent spasmodic coughing.

Can I Take Allergy Shots if I Am Pregnant?

Immunotherapy is considered safe and is generally maintained through pregnancy. Allergy injections contain the material that is absorbed into the body by breathing pollen and dust-laden air and can thus benefit the expectant mother by lessening the need for other medication. We usually reduce the maintenance dose and increase the frequency of the injections in order to minimize the risks of reactions. Immunotherapy should not be started during pregnancy, however; the risk of reaction is greatest during the initial period when the dose is increased.

Incidentally, women of child-bearing age should always let their allergists know when they are considering pregnancy. This will help in planning their treatment programs.

Which Diseases Are Helped by Immunotherapy?

The best results are obtained when allergy shots are given for pollen hayfever. Immunotherapy is also indicated for nasal and eye symptoms and asthma caused by house dust, molds, pollens, and animal danders.

When eczema is associated with pollen hayfever, it will sometimes improve with immunotherapy. The shots often make the eczema worse, however, and they must then be modified or stopped.

In very limited instances, hives are caused by inhalant allergens and desensitization may be helpful. Again, there are usually associated hayfever or asthma symptoms.

How Soon Do Allergy Shots Take Effect?

You can expect some improvement from immunotherapy after the maintenance dose has been reached. This may take three to six months, however, and the degree of improvement is variable. Some patients will soon experience good relief; others may not improve until a year or two later; but taking your shots regularly is most important.

Do Allergy Shots Always Work?

Allergy shots are beneficial in 80 to 90 percent of hayfever cases. Unfortunately, we cannot predict who will respond. Some patients experience complete relief whereas others at times still need to use medications. The allergic component of your asthma will also respond in a similar manner. Indeed, allergy shots can relieve your cat or pollen asthma, but the basic tendency to asthma will remain.

Reasons for failure include skipping injections, poor environmental control (cats and dust), and an unrecognized food allergy. The best results are achieved when properly prescribed antigen extracts are based on the correlation of appropriate skin test results with clinical symptoms.

How Often Do I Have to Take Allergy Shots?

Initially, allergy injections are given once or twice week. The dose is gradually increased toward the maintenance dosage. The small starting doses do not provide long-lasting protection, and adverse reactions are likely to occur if the interval between the increasing doses exceeds one to two weeks. In areas with short allergy seasons, allergy injections may be given prior to the pollen season. On the West Coast, allergy injections are usually given year round. Initially, shots are built up to a dose that is then maintained by injections every two to three weeks. After two years of treatment, they may be given every four weeks. Especially sensitive patients may require more frequent injections, and weekly injections are sometimes necessary for more than a year.

What Reactions Can I Expect From Allergy Shots?

In addition to the benefit from allergy shots, you may expect some transient reactions from immunotherapy since the extract contains what you are allergic to. This reaction usually amounts to only a small local area of redness and itching at the site of injection. A systemic reaction is always possible, however, involving sneezing, nasal discharge, watery eyes, coughing, wheezing, and even some sort of life-threatening reaction. This is the reason why we must start with a low dose then gradually "build you up" with each subsequent dose. In this manner you gradually become immune to the antigen so your body can tolerate the natural exposure.

Is the Dose Important?

Yes. Patients respond best to allergy shots when they receive the largest dose they can tolerate. Reaching the maximum requires an individualized program from your allergist.

The strength of the antigen is most commonly expressed as the ratio of the weight of pollen, for example, to the weight of water in which it is extracted. Pollen extracts are most commonly manufactured as 1:20 concentrates. Immunotherapy may begin with a concentration of 1:200,000 or 1:2,000,000. The maintenance dose should ideally be 1:200 or greater. Concentrations are sometimes expressed as a concentration of protein and in this system the maintenance dosage will be given from bottles labeled, for example, 10,000 protein/nitrogen units per milliliter (cc); the higher the number the more antigen in each vial.

What Happens if I Stop Allergy Shots for a Few Months?

If a long absence is necessary because of work or a vacation, the dose is reduced and is built back up at weekly intervals. The amount of reduction depends on your sensitivity, the previous maintenance dose, the length of time you have been on immunotherapy, and the time of your last shot. If you need year-round injections, a vacation should pose no problems. After two or three weeks, little or no adjustment should be necessary. If three or four months are missed, you will certainly need a dosage reduction and a build-up period of weekly treatments. We prepare extracts for our patients to take on extended vacations. The extracts can be administered by a local physician or aboard cruise ships by the ship's physician. Bon voyage!

How Long Will I Have to Take Allergy Shots?

Treatment should last a minimum of two to three years. Generally, children are more able to discontinue immunotherapy after this time. On the other hand, many adults must continue with allergy shots for a longer period.

If you wait to stop treatment until after two symptom-free years, your symptoms are less likely to recur.

Can Babies Receive Allergy Shots?

It is extremely unusual for an infant to develop allergy symptoms to pollens, dust, and molds during the first year or two of life. There has not really been much time for repeated exposure and increased sensitization, especially for seasonal pollens.

Skin testing can be done (and can be positive) at any age; however, the number of antigens to test for is much smaller during the first year or two, and not as many skin tests are necessary.

Allergy in the first two years of life is primarily related to foods, and the treatment is elimination, not allergy shots.

Can I Take Allergy Shots at Home?

Allergy injections contain a selection of antigens to which the patient is allergic. Each injection carries a risk of anaphylaxis and shock. The treatment schedule planned by your allergist should be individualized to minimize this risk. According to the National Institute of Health in a recent review of allergy and asthma, the patient should be observed for 15 to 30 minutes after each injection. The observer should have available the equipment and drugs necessary to treat shock and respiratory failure.

Getting injections at home is risky business. If you receive them in your physician's office, a serious reaction may be treated immediately. In rural areas, the benefits of immunotherapy may necessitate home injections, but in urban areas, the treatment should be given by your physician.

Do Allergy Shots Hurt?

Maybe a little. Injections are given with the smallest needles. Usually, sixteen drops of antigen or less is injected just under the skin. Itching and swelling may result, but discomfort from the injection itself is minimal. Even young children do not cry once they get over the fear of the initial injections.

How Expensive Are Allergy Shots?

Allergy shots range from $8.00 to $15.00 in the West and up to $25.00 in the East. This is the price for every allergy shot treatment whether your extract is divided into two or three shots or is given all in the same injection. Your cost during the first year could be anywhere from $400.00 to $1250.00. Thereafter, as the interval between injections increases, the cost should be less. The antigen extract used for your injection may be billed separately from the injections themselves, and this may cost about $100.00 per year.

The new venom extract for bee sting allergy is very expensive and the costs become much higher. This is reflected in the special charge for venom skin testing as well.

While you receive immunotherapy, your reactions are closely observed; your progress is monitored and necessary modifications of your dose and extract are made by trained nurses and your allergy specialist. The treatment visit includes careful record keeping and occasional prescription refills. Take the time to ask these professionals any questions you may have regarding your allergies.

8

Drug Allergies

Which Are the Most Allergenic Drugs?

Any drug may cause an allergic reaction, but penicillin is the most common cause of drug allergy. It has been widely studied, and skin testing can be done in order to confirm or rule out sensitivity. If you are truly allergic to penicillin, then you should also avoid ampicillin, amoxicillin, and the other penicillin-related antibiotics (Cloxacillin, etc.). Cephalosporins (keflex, etc.) are also related to penicillin; while the incidence is low, severe allergic reactions may occur in penicillin-allergic patients treated with keflex. It should be avoided, if possible.

Sulfa (sulfonamide) allergy is very severe and often results in a massive hivelike reaction called *erythema multiforme*. This antibiotic (Gantrisin, Gantanol) is widely used for urinary tract (bladder) infections. Currently, sulfa is often prescribed by pediatricians in combination with another antibiotic (the name of this combination is either Septra or Bactrim) for middle ear infections because of bacterial resistance to ampicillin and amoxicillin.

Tetracycline and erythromycin are frequently used broad-spectrum antibiotics. They have a much lower incidence of allergic potential; nevertheless, a patient may become sensitized. For this and other reasons these antibiotics should not be taken indiscriminantly.

Seizure medications—dilantin and phenobarbital—have caused prolonged allergic skin rashes and should always be considered possible causes.

How Do Drugs Cause Allergy?

Drugs cause allergic reactions in several ways. The allergy antibody IgE may be produced after a drug is taken. When the drug is taken again, the preformed antibody combines with the drug and the reaction occurs. The symptoms of anaphylaxis, whether mild or severe, can result. The spectrum of reaction ranges from mild itching to shock and death.

Other reactive antibodies may also be formed which cause such symptoms as easy bruising, hemorrhage, and anemia by destroying red blood cells.

A combination complex of the drug with the antibody can deposit in the tissues, causing lung and kidney damage. Fortunately, this reaction is rare.

Lymphocytes (a type of white blood cell) may become sensitized to drugs, causing skin rashes.

What Are the Side Effects of Drugs?

Many drugs have more than one effect. In the case of anti-histamines, relief from itching may be the desired effect, while drowsiness is a common side effect. Frequently, patients confuse side effects with allergies.

Some common drugs and their side effects are as follows:

Drug	Effect	Side Effects
Dilantin (diphenylhydantoin)	Prevents seizures	Overgrowth of gums
Aspirin	Relieves pain	Minute bleeding spots in the intestines
Erythromycin	Kills bacteria	Nausea
Antacids	Relieves pain of heartburn	Constipation or diarrhea
Birth control pills	Prevents ovulation	Increased incidence of stroke
Theophylline	Relieves wheezing	Irritability, stomachache, and headache
Chlorpheniramine	Dries allergic secretions	Drowsiness

Can Aspirin Cause Allergies?

Acetylsalicylic acid, commonly known as aspirin, can severely exacerbate asthma. It can also trigger hives and swelling of the larynx. Aspirin intolerance is present in at least 5 percent of asthmatics and in 1 percent of the general population.

An accurate history of aspirin intake accompanied by exacerbation of symptoms within thirty minutes is sufficient proof of aspirin intolerance. Marked improvement of symptoms after aspirin elimination is also sufficient proof. Clues of aspirin sensitivity include a persistent, watery, nasal discharge and nasal polyps.

If you have aspirin intolerance, all aspirin-containing products must be avoided. Read labels! Many over-the-counter pain and cold preparations such as Alka-Seltzer and Coricidin contain aspirin. Anti-inflammatory pain relieving medications, which are commonly used to treat arthritis and bursitis also aggravate intolerance in aspirin-sensitive patients; some of these are indomethacin (Indocin), phenylbutazone (Butazolidin), ibuprofen (Motrin), and tolmetin (Tolectin).

As many as one out of three aspirin-sensitive patients will experience difficulty after ingesting tartrazine yellow food coloring (FD&C No. 5). Tartrazine is found in many foods, particularly orange-flavored drinks, and is used to make some foods appear rich in eggs or butter. Oranges have even been injected with tartrazine for better color. Elimination and challenge testing with tartrazine may be indicated and should only be done under the supervision of your allergist.

Most aspirin-intolerant patients can tolerate acetaminophen (Tylenol, Liquiprin). This drug is useful in reducing fever and in treating pain, but it will not reduce the inflammation of arthritis or bursitis.

Can Skin Tests Be Used to Detect Drug Allergy?

Penicillin is the only drug that gives reliable skin test results. Special test materials are necessary: *both* a commercially available reagent and reagents prepared by your allergist must be used.

Skin tests may also be helpful in the preliminary evaluation of allergy to local anesthetics such as Xylocaine.

Can I Take Penicillin if I Am Allergic to It? What if I Really Need It?

Yes, you can take penicillin if it is absolutely necessary. Penicillin must be used in a severe life-threatening infection of the heart and in a few other rare instances. If there is penicillin allergy and no other drug can be used, a special "rush program" of desensitization will be carried out in a hospital intensive care unit. Multiple doses of penicillin are administered minutes apart until the strength needed for treatment is achieved without adverse side effects.

Can Dental Disclosing Tablets Cause Allergy?

Disclosing tablets contain a staining dye and are used to show plaque on teeth. Several kinds of disclosing tablets (Xpose, Red Cote) also contain the antibiotic erythromycin. Erythromycin is a potent photo-sensitizing drug when it is applied topically. When the tablet is dissolving in the mouth, the solution may come into contact with the lips. If the solution is not washed off, exposure to sunlight may result in a serious photoallergic reaction: swelling, blistering, and crusting of the lips.

How About Antibiotic Creams?

Antibiotic creams and ointments, such as Neosporin, may sensitize you and cause an allergic skin rash; their use should be limited. When large areas of skin are infected, treatment usually consists of orally administered penicillins or erythromycins.

Can I Become Allergic to My Allergy Medications?

Fortunately, allergy and asthma medications rarely cause drug allergies. Antihistamines may cause allergy when they are used on the skin. Reactions to antihistamines in eye drops are possible, but rarely occur.

Some over-the-counter allergy medications contain aspirin, which is frequently the cause of allergylike reactions. Allergy and asthma drugs may also contain offending coal-tar dyes such as tartrazine.

Does Codeine Cause Allergies?

When codeine is injected into normal skin, histamine is released from the mast cells in the skin and an itchy wheal and flare (hives) results. Some people are particularly sensitive to the action of codeine and experience generalized hives and itching when they take codeine by mouth. No allergy antibody is involved, however; this reaction is a serious *side effect* which may become progressively more severe. Codeine can also cause a true allergy reaction, but this is less frequent. Related drugs to be avoided include natural and synthetic narcotics, such as morphine, Demerol, and Talwin.

Can I Have Multiple Drug Allergies?

The frequency of drug allergies increases with age. Although patients do not develop allergies to all the drugs they take, allergy to two or three is not uncommon.

Can the Sun Cause Drug Reactions?

Yes. Some drugs, such as sulfa, tranquilizers (Thorazine), and some infrequently prescribed forms of tetracycline can make your skin exquisitely sensitive to the sun; even short exposure can result in severe sunburns.

In the presence of sunlight, some drugs can combine with proteins in your skin to form allergenic complexes. When you take the drug a second or third time and go out in the sun, a severe allergic skin rash can develop. Antiseptic agents (such as halogenated salicylamides) used in soaps may cause this reaction; sulfa drugs and thiazides (which are used for diuretic blood pressure control) may also be associated with this reaction. If you cannot avoid a drug to which you are photosensitive, you must use sun screens containing para-aminobenzoic acid (PABA) and avoid the sun.

Can One Develop a Cocaine Allergy?

Inhaling cocaine into the nose ("snorting") may result in typical allergylike symptoms: clear nasal discharge and conjunctival irritation with watery, itchy eyes. This is a common side effect of the drug, and prolonged use may result in destruction of the nasal septum.

Rare instances of true allergic reactions (anaphylaxis and asthma) have been reported.

Can I Prevent Drug Allergies?

You certainly can! Don't take antibiotics every time you might just have a viral infection such as the flu. "Shotgun" treatment may unnecessarily sensitize you to drugs that you may later need for a specific severe illness.

Good nutrition (chicken soup!) and rest are necessary for your immune system to fight infections effectively. But remember, of course, that antibiotics are required for many bacterial infections.

What Is G-6-P-D?

G-6-P-D, glucose-6-phosphate-dehydrogenase, is an enzyme necessary to maintain the integrity of red blood cells, that is, to keep them from leaking oxygen-carrying hemoglobin. A partial deficiency of this enzyme is an inherited condition, which most frequently affects black males. When G-6-P-D deficient people take certain drugs, such as Primaquine (for malaria) sulfa and phenacetin (in APCs — aspirin phenacetin caffein — empirin), their red blood cells break up and anemia results. Interestingly, eating fava beans can cause anemia, called *favism*, in those affected. This drug-caused anemia is nonallergic and is considered an idiosyncratic response.

What Is Erythema Multiforme?

Erythema multiforme is an exaggerated form of hives. The welts are large and have a "target" appearance: circular, red, and raised, with a clear area in the middle. The reaction is usually very severe and may progress to involve mucous membranes of the mouth, eyes, and genitals, and can be fatal despite intensive medical intervention.

Erythema multiforme most frequently results from an allergic reaction to sulfa. Common brand names to avoid, if you are allergic to sulfa, include Gantrisin, Gantanol, Septra,

Bactrim, and Azulfidine, as well as the "water pill," Diuril (thiazide). Many other drugs contain sulfa, and for this reason, if you have sulfa allergies you should always check with your physician or pharmacist to make sure that you are not prescribed drugs containing sulfa or related compounds.

Should I Wear a Medic Alert Bracelet or Necklace?

Some people should. A Medic Alert* necklace looks like a dogtag, and it will provide information about your medical condition and allergies in case of an emergency.

You should wear one if you have experienced a life-threatening reaction either to a drug such as penicillin or to a bee sting. Severe asthmatics, particularly children, should also wear one.

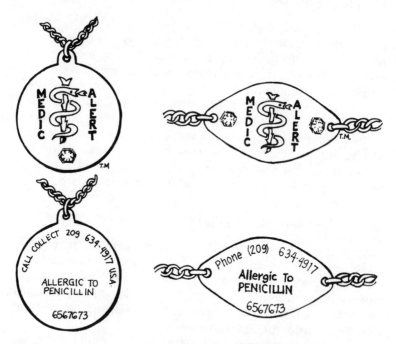

Medic Alert necklace (left) and bracelet (right).

*Medic Alert is a nonprofit foundation: P.O. Box 1009, Turlock, California 95380.

9

Controversial Issues – Behavioral and Body Systems

Should I Get a Room Ionizer?
Will Meditation Help My Allergy?
Are There Different Forms of Skin Testing?
What Is Sublingual Testing?
What Is the Neutralization Dose?
Should I Seek Acupuncture Treatment?
What Are Urine Shots?

What Is Anecdotal Evidence?

As physicians treating patients, we make many observations regarding our patients' disease and their responses to therapy. In medical school and specialty training, this accumulated knowledge contributes to our "clinical experience." Clinical experience transforms the student of medical texts into a physician. As we gain more experience, we can look for better methods of diagnosis and treatment. Often great advances have come from the observation or treatment of a single patient. In the 1800s Edward Jenner observed that milk maids who had been infected with cowpox were spared the ravages of smallpox. He had the courage to perform the first vaccination — to purposely give a mild disease (cowpox) in order to protect a young boy from smallpox. The World Health Organization feels that smallpox has now been eliminated as a threat to human health.

On the other hand, isolated observations may bear no relationship to the truth. We teach this to our children; feeling a bump on your head does not mean the sky is falling.

Patient testimonies do not prove that a medical treatment is effective or even safe. In medicine, we refer to the use of testimony to prove a new treatment as *anecdotal evidence;* it is interesting but not necessarily valid. Consider the case of the thymus irradiation, a popular "cure" for noisy breathing in babies, popular during the 1940s. This therapy was not only ineffective but also caused cancer of the thyroid.

Today, Doctor Jenner would need to follow the scientific and ethical standards of Jonas Salk and Albert Sabin in their development of polio vaccine. New diagnostic methods and treatments must be subjected to scientific study before they are used by the patient-consumer.

What Is the Placebo Effect?

A placebo is an inactive substance, drug, or treatment which is given to patients under the guise of being a genuine treatment. A beneficial clinical response often follows. This is known as the "placebo effect."

The placebo effect is well documented in medicine. Placebos can provide some symptomatic relief as much as 30 percent of the time. Patients' expectations and faith in therapy explain the effect.

If sugar pills were sold as aspirin, 30 percent of patients would report relief from their pain.

Do Some Individual Doctors Have Special Knowledge About Allergy?

There is no magic in medicine. You should be skeptical of any doctor who claims to have revolutionary and special methods of diagnosis or treatments. We occasionally hear of a doctor who is the only person in the community who has mastered a new and often dramatic system for healing. Some of these "cures" are the snake oil of today and are often uniquely expensive.

The Hippocratic oath requires that physicians teach their skills to others. Validated advances in therapy are rapidly accepted and widely used. Some examples of this are the treatment of diabetes with insulin and the current use of bee venoms for the treatment of bee allergy.

What Is Holistic Medicine? How Does It Relate to Allergy?

"Holistic" comes from the Greek word *holos*, which means whole. Simply, holistic medicine refers to the whole patient;

the psyche (mind) and body are one, an inseparable whole. In the extreme, holistic medicine teaches that if we lived in harmony in a pollution-free environment, we would be free of disease — in short, that we chose our own illnesses.

In the sense of "whole," good allergists are holistic practitioners. They realize that bad habits, such as cigarette smoking and poor nutrition, contribute to disease. They know that air pollution worsens asthma and is detrimental to the health of infants. A good allergist will help you understand your illness so you can better live with your allergies, and will teach you to alter your environment for better health.

Human beings can and will adapt to modern technology and its consequences; the masses of today cannot survive without it.

What Is Cerebral Allergy?

Cerebral allergy is a condition in which an individual shows a psychological reaction to environmental substances that are tolerated by nonallergic people. This reaction can express itself as difficulty in thinking or moving. There is no evidence that allergic reactions occur in the brain tissue, but changes in blood vessels — spasm or dilatation — are known to contribute to headache symptoms. So far, the evidence for cerebral or brain allergy is entirely anecdotal, and further research is necessary.

Can Food Allergy Cause Migraine Headaches?

Sometimes, the typical migraine headache responds to treatment with an elimination diet. Another type of headache that may clear with a food elimination is the "histamine" or "cluster" headache, which is usually located on only one side of the head and is associated with tearing from the eye on the same side.

The most common headache — the "tension headache" — may be caused by food allergy; in this case, a carefully followed regimen with elimination and challenge will often provide the important diagnostic clues. The cause of a "sinus headache" is usually the same food or inhalant factor — pollen, dust, mold — that is causing the stuffy nose and sneezing, which often accompany this type of headache.

Foods that should be investigated include, in order of frequency, chocolate, milk, corn, wheat, other grains, legumes, and foods with mold content. These may cause symptoms either alone or in combination.

The best indication that headaches can improve through dietary elimination is when the headaches occur as part of a total allergic presentation, with nasal allergy symptoms or asthma; nevertheless, it may indeed by the only complaint.

Sinus infection should always be considered. Before investigating possible food allergies, you should have your physician or a neurologist evaluate other possible serious causes of headache.

Can "Fad" Diets Affect My Health?

Yes. Fad diets such as macrobiotic, vegetarian, and fruitarian regimens often eliminate important and necessary nutrients. Some patients have experienced excessive weight loss leading to poor health. Vitamin and mineral deficiencies may also occur. There have been recent reports of rickets in children who are fed only "natural" unfortified foods and, at the same time, do not get adequate sunlight for vitamin D.

Should I Fast?

Fasting can be dangerous and is not advised for most persons. Such extreme elimination of all foods is not necessary for a careful investigation of food allergy, which can be accomplished with strict trial elimination of selected foods for three weeks at a time. Subsequent challenges with the eliminated foods confirms their roles as the cause of symptoms.

Rarely, a complete fast with the use of a nutrient substitute such as Vivonex might be of benefit. After totally eliminating all foods, the responsible allergen is identified when introduced into the diet. This *must* be done only under the close supervision of your physician.

Can Diet Help My Hyperactive Child?

Hyperactivity is rarely caused by food allergy. However, behavioral changes have been observed as a result from ingesting allergenic foods. These changes are known as the allergic-tension-fatigue syndrome. Your child may become more irritable, anxious, or excessively tired. The appearance of facial pallor, dark circles around the eyes, and complaints about stomach aches and headaches are all part of this syndrome. Symptoms are improved by proper elimination diet of offending foods.

Controlled studies have shown that preservatives and food colorings only rarely cause hyperactivity.

Can Sugar Cause Allergy?

Sugars do not cause allergy. Chemically, sugars are called *saccharides*. Glucose and fructose are found in fruits and vegetables; they are called simple sugar units or *monosaccharides*. Fructose is the very sweet sugar found in honey. Sucrose, the sugar found in cane and beets, is a compound of glucose and fructose and is termed a *disaccharide*. Lactose, the sugar of milk, is a combination of glucose and a unique milk sugar, galactose. Milk sugar and sucrose must be broken down to the simple monosaccharides before they can be absorbed from the intestines.

A current fad considers honey (fructose) to be natural and refined or purified sucrose from sugar cane as unnatural. Actually, both are equally natural. When you eat cane sugar, the body absorbs the digested products, glucose and fructose.

When many sugar units are joined together by plants or bacteria, starch and polysaccharides are formed. Only certain polysaccharides are commonly found in the cell walls of bacteria and can act as antigens, causing the body to form antibodies. Starch and other polysaccharides have not been shown to cause the formation of allergy antibodies; neither have the mono- or disaccharides. Thus, sugar and other polysaccharides play no role in allergy.

Corn syrup is often used as a sweetener, and this "sugar" has indeed been shown to cause allergy.

Can Vitamins Help My Allergy?

Vitamins work to "cure" and prevent colds by protecting mucous membranes from damage caused by viral infection.

Some cold symptoms associated with or which mimic allergies can be controlled with large vitamin doses, but the real value of this treatment has not been conclusively demonstrated.

What Is Bee Pollen?

Bee pollen is pollen extracted from the surface of bee extremities. It is high in protein content and is sold in health food stores. Some bee pollens share similar components with the allergenic pollen that we breathe. Severe allergic attacks and even anaphylaxis have been reported in pollen-sensitive individuals after they ingest bee pollen.

Can I Be Allergic to Chlorinated Water?

Chlorine is not an allergen. Therefore, it cannot induce new allergies. Chlorine can, however, provoke symptoms that mimic allergies. It can irritate your eyes, nasal mucosa, and eczema skin lesions whenever you swim in improperly chlorinated water. It can even make you sneeze!

What About Ginseng?

An ancient Chinese monk once commented, "Ginseng will convey you with the speed of the wind to the grotto of eternal spring. It will give your loins twofold, nay, tenfold vigor, anchor your teeth more firmly, and increase the keenness of your sight."

This prized herb, which is extracted from a root of the plant panax, has been used by the Chinese for over 4000 years. It is used to revitalize as well as to treat asthma and other disorders such as diabetes and sexual impotence.

Scientists have studied the herb and found that it contains several active pharmacologic substances (panaxin, panax acid, and pancen) which increase body metabolism and stimulate a number of organs such as the heart and nervous system.

There are different types of ginseng: *Panax quinquefolia* (American) and *Panax ginseng* (Korean, Chinese). The Eastern type is rare and very expensive. The American type is more plentiful and less expensive, but it is less potent.

What About Chamomile Tea?

Drinking chamomile tea is a popular folk cure for respiratory illness and flu in Western European cultures. Interestingly, chamomile is in the ragweed family and serious allergic reactions to it have been reported. If you have a ragweed allergy, you should not drink chamomile tea.

Is Arthritis an Allergy?

Many causes of arthritis have been discovered, and allergy is not among them. Patients who are suffering from severe allergies may feel general sickness or malaise and their joints may ache, but they do not have any long-lasting disability or deformity.

What Is Petrochemical Allergy?

Petrochemicals are potentially potent toxins; that is, in various concentrations, they can cause illness in all people. Petrochemicals are the various hydrocarbons distilled from petroleum. The fumes of these chemicals, such as gasoline, can cause headaches, malaise, and nausea. In high concentrations they can be fatal. Altered immune reactions (allergy) to these substances have not, however, been reported.

Why Do Hairsprays, Insect Sprays, and Air Fresheners Make My Allergy Worse?

Hairsprays contain chemical irritants which trigger the allergic response. Neither hairsprays nor the chemicals in air fresheners and cleaning preparations cause allergies as such. They can cause your allergic symptoms of nasal congestion or wheezing to flare up, and you are more susceptible to these irritants precisely because you are allergic; your allergic mucous membranes are far more prone to react than those of a nonallergic individual.

Should I Get a Room Ionizer?

The ionizer generates charged particles called *negative ions* into the air; these negative ions bind onto particulate matter, thus forming larger precipitates; the larger and heavier particles then settle to the ground.

This sounds like a good idea, but room ionizers have not been proven beneficial in allergies. They may remove allergenic particles such as dust and pollens from a small area surrounding the machine itself, but not provide sufficiently wide environmental control.

Will Meditation Help My Allergy?

It may help. Meditation resolves psychic and physical stress, factors which definitely aggravate your allergic status. This therapy has been practiced for hundreds of years by scholars and mystics in Europe and India.

Airway resistance in asthma and vascular dilatation in allergic rhinitis are partially under the control of the autonomic (nonvoluntary) nervous system. Meditation with subsequent central nervous system stimulation and inhibition may modify this autonomic balance with symptomatic relief.

Are There Different Forms of Skin Testing?

The most widely used and accepted form of skin testing is the scratch technique using concentrates of different allergen extracts. This may be followed with some selected intradermal tests which utilize a weaker dilution. Treatment is based on positive tests that have significance in terms of the clinical history. Allergy shots are started at a weak dilution then progress slowly to stronger dilutions as they are tolerated.

There are other techniques which utilize varying diluations of the same allergen with intradermal injections. Results are interpreted with regard to the specific size and quality of the wheal formations in order to establish the correct dose for treatment. Future adjustment of the dose is often necessary. This variation of diagnosis and treatment has not been demonstrated to be effective by controlled studies, even though anecdotal reports of efficacy by reliable and experienced practitioners exist.

What Is Sublingual Testing?

Sublingual testing is an attempt to diagnose allergies by provoking allergy symptoms. The method involves placing drops of diluted allergenic material under the tongue. A positive test is reported when the patient states that symptoms have developed or when the observer notes difficulty in breathing, random eye movements, or lethargy. This method has not yet been tested according to objective and reproducible parameters such as lung or pulmonary function tests or measurements of nasal swelling through airway flow rates. In contrast, skin tests provide a measurable reaction in the skin whose accuracy has been proven.

What Is the Neutralization Dose?

Some practitioners claim that allergic symptoms can be turned off or "neutralized" by administering a dilute concentration of the allergen. This dose is injected or placed as a drop under the tongue (sublingual).

The idea is appealing, but no controlled studies have shown it to be effective. In fact, recent studies have shown the opposite to be true; the best relief occurs when patients have become desensitized by receiving progressively larger doses of antigen — the higher the maintenance dose the greater the relief.

Should I Seek Acupuncture Treatment?

Medications are far more effective than acupuncture in the treatment of asthma; acupuncture has helped some asthmatics, however, and has been successfully used as an adjunct therapy in selected cases. The therapeutic effect of acupuncture treatment is short-termed.

What Are Urine Shots?

Believe it or not, some attempt has been made to treat allergies by injecting patients with their own urine. We can't imagine the rationale for this procedure. Moreover, it is known that experimental rabbits injected with their own urine will develop severe kidney disease. *Don't be a guinea pig!*

10

Where Do I Go From Here?

Can I Diagnose Allergies Myself?

Any keen observer can! You can start by focusing on conditions and situations that may aggravate your allergy symptoms. For example, if your symptoms are worse indoors, then you should suspect house dust or mold allergy; nighttime and early morning sneezing attacks are suggestive of house dust allergy and of mold allergy, especially in moist and sheltered environments. Do you notice that symptoms are worse when you come home to your dog or cat and improve when you leave? Are you symptom free outdoors? Did you check your pillows for feathers?

If your hayfever is always worse on the golf course, then grass pollen is the most likely offender.

Which Allergies Can I Treat by Myself?

The best treatment of allergy always includes self-help. Avoidance is consistently the preferred form of therapy. If you are sensitive, don't visit parks and roll on the grass during April and May — and no unnecessary weekend trips to the country during these months. If your sneezing, watery eyes, and wheezing are worse around dogs and cats, put them outside and don't visit homes with indoor pets.

Adequate rest — sometimes just an extra hour of sleep — and good nutrition are most important. These measures are often very helpful.

Take an antihistamine like Chlor-Trimeton if you are in an unavoidable allergic circumstance. It may be all that is necessary to ward off disturbing and uncomfortable symptoms.

How Can I Control My Environment?

FOR HOUSE DUST

The bedroom should be given first priority because you spend approximately six to ten hours a day breathing the air in that room.

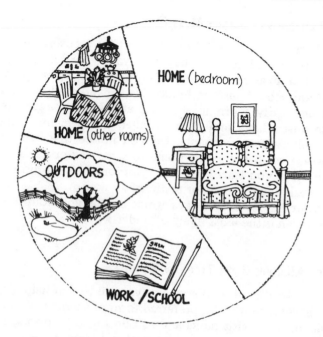

Proportion of day spent in different environments.

1. Cover *all* mattresses and boxsprings in your bedroom with zippered plastic or canvas encasings. The stronger canvas encasings can be obtained from Allergen-Proof Encasings, Inc., 1450 East 363rd Street, Eastlake, Ohio 44094.
2. Vacuum the mattresses and areas around and underneath the beds, including the closets, at least once every week; daily wet mopping of floors is very effective.
3. Bare floors and windows without draperies are best, although small washable synthetic rugs and curtains may be used.
4. Remove upholstered furniture, stuffed toys, books and bookcases, and other dust-collecting items from the bedroom. Dacron or foam rubber may be substituted for the potential dust-producing material that is commonly found in stuffed toys. It takes only a moment of sewing.

5. An allergic individual should also avoid feathers; check your pillows, comforters, and clothing.

FOR MOLDS

1. An ordinary chlorine bleach, such as Clorox, is effective for eradicating molds and mildew. Lysol is also a good household cleansing agent.
2. Recognize "hot spots" where molds are most likely to accumulate. Damp and sheltered environments encourage mold growth. These areas include:
   - bathroom and kitchen sink areas; behind refrigerators, around showers, tubs, toilets; cabinets and floor areas
   - mattresses and boxsprings, especially the underside surfaces
   - walls, especially old wallpaper and wallpaper behind furniture, desks, bookcases (use mold-inhibiting paints)
   - under porches and basement areas
   - closets
   - garden and yard areas (piles of leaves)
   - indoor household plants (remove them from the bedroom)
   - washing machine area
   - wicker baskets, carpet padding, humidifiers, air conditioners

Are Natural Foods Important?

Yes. Some patients experience allergic symptoms after eating foods containing colorings, preservatives, and other additives. Foods you prepare yourself will not contain these possible offenders. A strict trial elimination diet that uses only natural foods may be helpful.

If your symptoms subside with a natural food diet, you will be able to buy good products in most supermarkets. But remember, foods labeled "natural" or "organic" can still contain a variety of additives; take the time to read labels carefully.

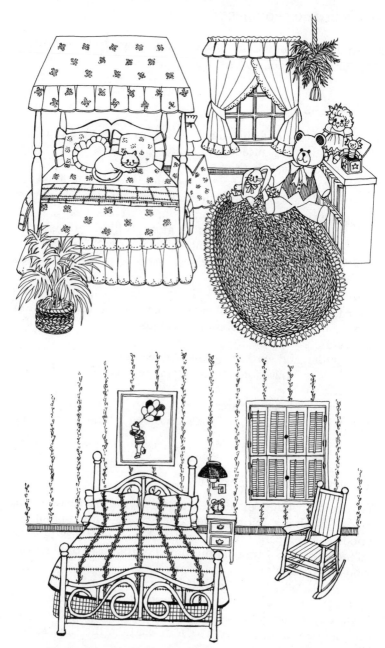

Allergenic room (top) and nonallergenic room (bottom).

Will an Air Filter Help?

Breathing cleaner air has given many hayfever and asthma sufferers good relief. This can be achieved by installing air-cleaning machines and special filters.

Choosing the right air cleaner or filter is important. High efficiency particulate air filters (HEPA) have been demonstrated to be effective in trapping most airborne allergens, such as pollen, mold, and house dust particles. The filter material is made of tiny glass fibers interfolded to allow the entrapment of small particles as the air is filtered through it. This filter is an important component in several commercial air cleaners. Prices for an air cleaner vary according to the size and model The air cleaner can be adjusted to any room, although the bedroom should deserve first priority. An average bedroom air cleaner will cost around $300.00.

The second type of air cleaner utilizes an electrostatic precipitator device which magnetically traps charged particles. A major disadvantage of such a system is that some models emit ozone. Ozone levels at 0.3 ppm (parts per million by volume of air) can precipitate coughing and choking and can make your asthma worse. Lower levels cause nasal and eye irritation.

An air cleaner should be rented first to evaluate its effectiveness. Stores will often credit the customer's rental costs toward the purchase cost, which is tax-deductible for medical expenses.

Should I Take a Vacation During Pollen Season?

Super idea! You may have trouble deducting it as a medical expense, but a vacation during a short two- or three-week pollen season could be a very effective treatment for your allergies. The difficulty with this includes the time you may have to be away and the distance that may be necessary to travel. You may also just trade your ragweed symptoms for other severe pollen or mold allergies in the vacation area. In fact, for most patients this is not practical.

Immunotherapy with allergy shots will provide relief 90 percent of the time. This is far more reliable and realistic than island hopping all year.

How Can I Build Up My Wind?

You can "build up your wind" with an exercise program that becomes progressively more strenuous. If such a program is followed regularly, your breathing will become less labored with activities and exertion.

We encourage asthmatic patients to participate in sports activities, especially swimming. Other aerobic exercises, such as jogging and long walks, ballet, and jazz exercise, are excellent. You can also benefit from "pumping iron" and other regulated weight programs such as Nautilus.

Will Breathing Exercises Help My Asthma?

Breathing exercises teach efficient breathing and relaxation; you will learn the technique of diaphragmatic breathing — using the diaphragm to take in more air.

These techniques are not necessary for most asthmatics but are helpful for panic-stricken children who have frequent attacks.

Breathing exercises should not and cannot be a substitute for medications.

Which Over-the-Counter Drugs Are O.K. to Use?

The safest over-the-counter allergy drugs are plain antihistamines, such as Chlor-Trimeton. This may provide some relief from hayfever as well as hives. The combination antihistamine-decongestants like ARM may also be used, but you should seek a physician's supervision if you have a history of other medical problems such as high blood pressure.

Prescription medicine is often necessary for severe symptoms. If you are wheezing with asthma, you may indeed get temporary relief with Primatene Mist, but the best drugs are only available by prescription.

At What Point Should I See an Allergist?

When your symptoms are inadequately controlled in spite of all your efforts to self-diagnose and treat yourself, you should seek medical advice. Your physician can help you evaluate the extent of the problem. Allergy consultation with an allergist may be necessary to detect allergens that may have escaped your notice and to plan the best treatment.

How Do I Choose an Allergist?

The best way to choose an allergist is by first asking your primary care physician or the local medical society for a referral. Then make inquiries with other physicians as well as community professionals and friends. Finally, you might ask the office receptionist by phone regarding board certification and training in allergy, as well as medical school faculty appointments, and activity in local allergy societies. Positive replies to all the above do not always guarantee success in your choice; nevertheless, they are the most helpful guidelines.

Certification by the American Board of Allergy and Immunology currently requires completion of a two-year postgraduate fellowship in allergy and immunology. After training, a young physician must pass a difficult qualifying examination which encompasses all phases of allergy and immunology including asthma and other chest diseases, aerobiology, and skin disorders.

Also, interpersonal relationships, while intangible, are always important. If you cannot communicate with your allergist, a change is necessary.

Will Insurance Provide for My Allergy Care?

If your insurance covers office visits as well as hospitalizations, you are probably covered for allergy. Allergy care thus comes under the same category as any other medical problem such as high blood pressure. It is not a routine visit for a check-up.

How Much Will Allergy Consultation Cost?

The cost of a complete allergy consultation with necessary skin tests may run up to $400.00.

The consultation with a detailed history and physical examination is the most important and valuable part of your allergy evaluation and can vary in cost from $50.00 to $150.00, depending on the part of the country and the complexity of the problem. Complete skin testing usually costs around $200.00. If you are only concerned about a limited problem such as cats and dogs, your allergist will only need to perform a limited number of skin tests; this should not cost more than $50.00. Additional pulmonary function breathing tests (spirometry) should be done on all patients with asthma, and this usually costs about $75.00. You may want to inquire by telephone about these component fees as well as the total cost.

Remember, it is impossible to compare the value of personal professional services — variables include the availability of the allergist, the allergist's qualifications, and the time spent with you, the patient.

Glossary

Adrenalin (epinephrine): A powerful hormone that relaxes bronchial muscles, stimulates the heart, and is necessary for the treatment of severe allergic reactions

Allergen: A protein substance that causes the formation of allergy antibodies and subsequently triggers the allergic response

Anaphylaxis: A severe and immediate allergic reaction

Angioedema: Swelling of various body parts, especially around the eyes and lips

Antibody: A serum protein which fights infection or causes allergy

Antihistamine: The most commonly used drug for allergies; blocks histamines and thereby prevents allergic response

Bronchitis: Inflammation or infection of the bronchial tubes in the lungs

Bronchodilator: Medication that relaxes the spasm of the bronchial tubes in asthma

Celiac disease: Diarrhea and malabsorption of food caused by intolerance to gluten, a protein of wheat, rye, oats, and barley

Conjunctivae: The inner linings of the eyelid and the covering of the eyeball

Cortisone: An important steroid used to treat severe allergic reactions

Dander: Flecks of skin which are shed by pets and people; a frequent cause of allergy and food for mites

Eczema: An itchy and dry skin rash, often caused by allergy

Eosinophils: White blood cells that increase in number in allergic conditions; also found in bronchial tubes and nasal secretions

Histamine: A chemical substance, released by mast cells, that causes the allergic symptoms of itching, swelling, and bronchial spasms

Immunotherapy: Treatment of allergies by injection of allergens (allergy shots)

Intradermal testing: Allergy skin tests performed by injection of allergens into the skin

Lymphocytes: White blood cells that produce antibodies and regulate the immune response

Mast cells: Cells containing histamine and slow-reacting substance of anaphylaxis (SRSA); found in the mucous membranes, bronchial tubes, and skin

Mold: A minute fungus — for instance, mildew — which causes allergy by producing airborne spores

Mucous membranes: The moist linings of the mouth, nose, and other parts of the respiratory, digestive, and reproductive systems

Slow-reacting substance of anaphylaxis (SRSA): The most important chemical mediator of asthma; produced by the bronchial mast cells

Steroids: Hormones, such as cortisone, that regulate body functions and are produced by the endocrine glands

Tartrazine: A coal-tar dye that can cause asthma and hives; used as a yellow food coloring (FD&C No. 5)

Urticaria: Hives or welts

Venom: The poison of stinging insects which contains allergens

Index